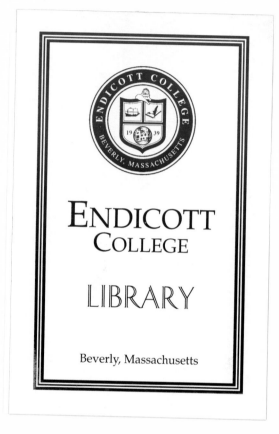

ENDICOTT
COLLEGE

LIBRARY

Beverly, Massachusetts

Anabolic Steroids
and Sports

Anabolic Steroids and Sports

A Selective Bibliography with Annotations

Compiled by
Ellen R. Paterson

The Whitston Publishing Company
Troy, New York
1991

Copyright 1991
The Whitston Publishing Company

Library of Congress Catalog Card Number 90-83684

ISBN 0-87875-389-3

Printed in the United States of America

Contents

Preface

This publication was compiled for athletes, parents, coaches, physicians, teachers, librarians and the general public as a guide to the most recent important information on anabolic steroids and sports published in both popular and professional literature. General and professional overview articles are listed and sometimes annotated as well as articles on specific topics and/or users such as: Ben Johnson, Children and Adolescents, Education and Counseling, HGH and Somatotropin, Side Effects, Testing and Drug Enforcement, Training Alternatives, and Women.

Over 600 references to articles, books, book chapters, films, pamphlets, theses, ERIC and government documents published between 1979 and 1990 are listed in this bibliography. Some 200 references have been annotated and these are concentrated in the topical areas rather than the general/popular articles whose titles are often descriptive of their content.

Books, book chapters, films, pamphlets, theses, and documents are listed alphabetically by author or editor. Periodical literature is listed under appropriate headings and arranged alphabetically by title under each subject. References that treat more than one topic are not repeated, but appear once in the most appropriate section. A glossary has been provided to explain frequently used terms and colloquial expressions. Some 350 first-cited authors and editors are listed in an author index. A brief subject index is also provided. Animal studies and articles in a foreign language have been excluded.

The following indexes and abstract services have been searched in compiling this volume:

Education Index
ERIC on CD-ROM and DIALOG file 1
General Science Index
Index Medicus and Medline or DIALOG file 154
Index to Legal Periodicals
Magazine and Newspaper Indexes and DIALOG files 47 and 111
Nursing and Allied Health or DIALOG file 218
Physical Education Index
PsycLIT on CD-ROM
Readers' Guide to Periodical Literature
Social Sciences Index on CD-ROM
SOCIOFILE on CD-ROM
Sport Discus and DIALOG file 48

Ellen R. Paterson (B.S., R.N., M.L.S., C.A.S.)
Reference Bibliographer for the Sciences and Health
State University Of New York College at Cortland

List of Journals Cited

Acta Dermato-Venereologica
Acta Endocrinologica
Acta Medica Hungarica
Aerobics
American Pharmacy
American Family Physician
American Health
American Journal of Cardiology
American Journal of Clinical Hypnosis
American Journal of Clinical Nutrition
American Journal of Dermatopathology
American Journal of Diseases of Children
American Journal of Hospital Pharmacy
American Journal of Nursing
American Journal of Psychiatry
American Journal of Sports Medicine
American School Board Journal
American School and University
Annals of Sports Medicine
Annual Review of Pharmacology and Toxicology
Arena Review
Athletic Business
Athletic Director and Coach
Athletic Training
Athletics
Audible
Australian Family Physician
Australian Journal of Science and Medicine in Sport
Badminton Now
Bicycling
Biomedical and Environmental Mass Spectrometry
British Journal of Sports Medicine
British Medical Journal
CAHPER Journal
Canadian Athletic Therapists Association Journal
Canadian Journal of Applied Sport Sciences
Canadian Pharmaceutical Journal
Capital University Law Review
Christian Science Monitor
Chronicle of Higher Education
Clinical Chemistry

Clinical Orthopaedics and Related Research
Clinical Pharmacy
Clinical Psychologist
Clinics in Sports Medicine
Coaching Women's Basketball
Comprehensive Therapy
Current Health
Delaware Medical Journal
Dickinson Law Review
Drake Law Review
Economist
Electroencephalography and Clinical Neurophysiology
Emergency Medicine
European Journal of Applied Physiology and Occupational Physiology
Excel
Executive Fitness
FDA Consumer
FIEP Bulletin
First Aider
Flex
Futurist
Handball
Hastings Center Report
Health Education
Health Letter
Hospital Formulary
Howard Law Journal
Indiana Law Journal
International Journal of Cardiology
International Journal of Sport Psychology
International Journal of Sports Medicine
International Journal of the History of Sport
Iron Man
JAMA : Journal of the American Medical Association
Jet
John Marshall Law Review
Journal of Adolescent Health Care
Journal of Biosocial Science Supplement
Journal of the American Academy of Dermatology
Journal of Applied Physiology: Respiratory, Environmental and Exercise
      Physiology
Journal of the Arkansas Medical Society
Journal of Clinical Endocrinology and Metabolism
Journal of Clinical Pathology
Journal of Clinical Psychiatry
Journal of Drug Education
Journal of Drug Issues
Journal of Hand Surgery
Journal of the Medical Association of Georgia
Journal of Nuclear Medicine and Allied Science
Journal of Osteopathic Sports Medicine
Journal of Physical Education, Recreation and Dance
Journal of the South Carolina Medical Association
Journal of Sport History
Journal of Sports Medicine and Physical Fitness
Journal of Steroid Biochemistry
Lancet

Legal Memorandum
Los Angeles Times
Maclean's
Medicine and Science in Sports and Exercise
Modern Athlete and Coach
Muscle and Fitness
Muscular Development
National Federation News
National Strength and Conditioning Association Journal
New England Journal of Medicine
New Scientist
New York Times
New Zealand Journal of Sports Medicine
Newsweek
Nurse Practitioner
Omni
Patient Care
Pediatric Annals
Pediatric Clinics of North America
Pediatric Nursing
Pediatrics
Pepperdine Law Review
Personnel Journal
Pharos
Physician Assistant
Physician and Sports Medicine
Plastic and Reconstructive Surgery
Postgraduate Medicine
Powerlifting USA
Psychology Today
Reader's Digest
Recent Studies in Cancer Research
Research Quarterly for Exercise and Sport
Runner's World
Saturday Evening Post
Saturday Night
Scandinavian Journal of Sports Sciences
Scholastic Coach
Scottish Medical Journal
Seminars in Adolescent Medicine
Sociology and Social Research
Southern California Law Review
Soviet Sports Review
Sport Talk
Sporting News
Sports Illustrated
Sports Medicine
Sports Medicine Bulletin
Sportsmedicine Digest
Sports: Science Periodical on Research and Technology
Strength and Health
Swimming World and Junior Swimmer
Technology Review
Texas Coach
Thurgood Marshall Law Review
Time
Track and Field Quarterly Review

Track Technique
U. S. News and World Report
Ultrasport
University of Florida Law Review
University of Kansas Law Review
University of Toronto Faculty of Law Review
USA Today
Wall Street Journal
Washington Post
Weightlifters Newsletter
Women and Health
Women's Sports and Fitness
Wrestling USA
Your Health and Fitness

Books, Films, Pamphlets, Theses

Alen, M. "Androgenic-anabolic steroid effects on endocrinology in adult male athletes" in SCANDINAVIAN CONFERENCE IN SPORTS MEDICINE, 2, OSLO 1986. AN UPDATE ON SPORTS MEDICINE. . . . Strommen: Syntex, 1987. pp. 145-152.

"American College of Sports Medicine position stand on the use of anabolic-androgenic steroids in sports" in DRUGS AND PERFORMANCE IN SPORTS, edited by R. H. Strauss. Philadelphia: W. B. Saunders, 1987. pp. 199-209.

American College of Sports Medicine. POSITION STANDS AND OPINION STATEMENTS, 7th edition. Indianapolis: The College, 1987. 38pp.

American Medical Association. DRUG EVALUATIONS, 6th edition. Chicago: The Association, 1986
Androgens and anabolic steroids are discussed on pp. 675 to 687.

Asken, Michael J. DYING TO WIN: ATHLETE'S GUIDE TO SAFE AND UNSAFE DRUGS IN SPORTS. Washington, D.C.: Acropolis Books, 1988.
Anabolic steroids are discussed on pages 89-93, their positive and negative effects and the position of the American College of Sports Medicine.

Bach, Julie S. DRUG ABUSE: OPPOSING VIEWPOINTS. St. Paul: Greenhaven Press, 1988.

Berger, Gilda. DRUG TESTING. New York: Watts, 1987. 63 pp.
This book includes discussion of mandatory testing for college athletes.

Brown, T. C., and C. Benner. "Nonmedical use of drugs in sports" in PRINCIPLES OF SPORTS MEDICINE, edited by W. N. Scott. Baltimore: Williams and Wilkins, 1984. pp. 32-39.

BULKING UP: THE DANGER OF STEROIDS. Van Nuys, CA: Aims Media, 1990. $395.00 video; $495.00 16mm.
Narrated by Bruce Jenner, this video gives an excellent detailed description and analysis of the dangers of anabolic steroids.

Cairo, R. J. ANABOLIC STEROIDS AND THEIR RELATIONSHIP TO LIVER FUNCTIONS (dissertation). Eugene, Oregon: Microform Publications, 1987. 2 microfiches. 109 fr.

Canadian Track and Field Association. THE DEVELOPING ATHLETES' HANDBOOK. Ottawa: The Track and Field Association, 1986. 99pp.

CHAMPIONS AT ANY PRICE. Columbus: Exceed Sports Nutritionals, 1988. Videotape 22 min. $10.
This film presents physiological and psychological problems associated with steroid use.

Colby, H. D., and P. A. Longhurst. "Fate of anabolic steroids in the body" in DRUGS, ATHLETES AND PHYSICIAL PERFORMANCE, edited by J. A. Thomas. New York: Plenum Medical Book Company, 1988. pp. 11-30.

Committee on Sports Medicine, American Academy of Pediatrics: SPORTS MEDICINE: HEALTH CARE FOR YOUNG ATHLETES, edited by N. J. Smith. Elkgrove Village, Illinois. American Academy of Pediatrics, 1987.
Chapter 13 "Drugs and Athletics" pp. 176-183, discusses doping and specifically steroids on pp. 181-182 and reviews adverse side effects.

CURRENT MEDICAL DIAGNOSIS AND TREATMENT. Norwalk, Connecticut: Appleton and Lange, 1989. p. 761
Anabolics (sex steroids) briefly discussed.

Dawson, Tim R. EDUCATOR'S GUIDE TO THE LITERATURE DEALING WITH THE RATIONALE FOR STEROID USE, EFFECTS THEY HAVE ON BODY COMPOSITION AND PERFORMANCE, WITH SOLUTIONS TO PREVENTING STEROID ABUSE IN YOUTH [dissertation]. Indiana University at South Bend, 1989. 31 pp.
This study provides information about steroids and recommends programs to educators and coaches who are involved with educating students about steroid abuse.

Deighan, W. P., compiler. TEAM UP FOR DRUG PREVENTION WITH AMERI-CA'S YOUNG ATHLETES. Washington, D. C.: Drug Enforcement Administration, Department of Justice, 1986. 29pp.

DiPasquale, M. G. DRUG USE AND DETECTION IN AMATEUR SPORTS. Warkworth, Ontario: M.G.D. Press, 1984.

Dolan, E. F. DRUGS IN SPORTS. New York: Franklin Watts, 1986.

Donohoe, T. and N. Johnson. FOUL PLAY: DRUG ABUSE IN SPORTS. New York: Basil Blackwell, 1986.
Anabolic steroids (chapter 3, pp. 38-65) are covered in terms of physiology, research study on effectiveness, and detection. Steroid abuse is mentioned in other chapters such as "drugs and the female athlete (chapter 4).

DRUG TESTING. Reston, Virginia: National Association of Secondary School Principals, 1987. 9pp.

Dye, C. ANABOLIC STEROIDS. Phoenix: Do it Now Foundation, 1989. 4pp.
This is a good general introduction to the use of steroids, doping and stacking, placebo effect, health risks, and superstar syndrome. Human Growth Hormone is also discussed. William Taylor is the sports medicine consultant.

Dyment, P. G. "Stimulant drug use by young athletes" in COMMON PROBLEMS IN PEDIATRIC SPORTS MEDICINE, edited by N. J. Smtih. Chicage: Year Book Medical Publishers, 1989. pp. 125-130.

ENHANCING PERFORMANCE: THE ROLE OF NUTRITION IN ATHLETICS.
Columbus: Exceed Sports Nutritionals, 1988. Videotape. $10.16 min.
This videotape includes discussion of four nutritional periods considered critical for peak performance.

FOR COACHES ONLY: HOW TO START A DRUG PREVENTION PROGRAM.
Washington, D. C.: Drug Enforcement Administration, Department of Justice, 1986. 17pp.

Gaines, C. and G. Butler. IRON SISTERS: WORLD OF WOMEN'S BODYBUILD-ING. New York: Simon and Schuster, 1984.

—. PUMPING IRON II: THE UNPRECEDENTED WOMAN. New York: Simon and Schuster, 1984.

Ganong, R. UNIVERSITY OF MIAMI HURRICANE FOOTBALL TEAM OFF-SEASON STRENGTH TRAINING PROGRAM. Coral Gables: Miami University, 1983. 121pp.

George, A. J. "Anabolic Steroids" in DRUGS IN SPORT, edited by D. R. Mottram. Champaign, Illinois: Human Kinetics, 1988. pp. 59-78.

Gleeson, G. THE GROWING CHILD IN COMPETITIVE SPORT. Toronto: Hodder and Stoughton, 1986.
This book has chapters on strength training and endurance training (pp. 15-43).

Goldman, B. DEATH IN THE LOCKER ROOM: STEROIDS AND SPORTS. South Bend, Indiana: Icaus, 1984.
This is an often cited reference on drugs and sports with chapters on women athletes and physicial effects of drugs on athletes. Position statements on anabolic steroids are in the extensive appendices.

—. INTERNATIONAL FEDERATION OF BODYBUILDERS. Montreal. 1981. 35 pp.

—. THE "E" FACTOR. New York: Morrow, 1988.
This book covers nutritional ergogenic aids, longevity and the athelete, drugs, hormones, drug detection techniques, and evaluation of equip-ment and training systems in parts 1 and 2. Part 3 introduces sports psy-chology, subliminal testing, biofeedback, pulse monitoring and elec-tronics in the treatment of sports injuries. Position papers on anabolic steroids included in the extensive appendices.

Hackman, R. M. "Leading edge: nutrition and athletic performance" in SPORT, HEALTH AND NUTRITION, edited by F. I. Katch. Champaign, Ill.: Human Kinetics Publishers, 1986. pp. 3-10.

Harris, Jonathan. DRUGGED ATHLETES: CRISIS IN AMERICAN SPORTS. New York: Four Winds, 1987.

Hatfield, Frederick C. ANABOLIC STEROIDS: WHAT KIND AND HOW MANY. Madison, Wisconsin: Fitness System, 1982.

—. BODYBUILDING: A SCIENTIFIC APPROACH. Chicago: Contemporary Books, 1984. 276 pp.

—. POWER: A SCIENTIFIC APPROACH: ADVANCED MUSCLEBUILDING TECHNIQUES FOR EXPLOSIVE STRENGTH. Chicago: Contemporary, 1989.
> Hatfield describes the benefits of anabolic steroids, methods of use, stacking and other techniques for strength training.

Haymes, E. M. "Nutrition and ergogenic aids" in PHYSICAL ACTIVITY AND WELL-BEING, edited by V. Seefeldt. Reston, Virginia: American Alliance for Health, Physical Education, Recreation and Dance, 1986. pp.237-273.

Hervey, G. R. "What Are the Effects of Anabolic Steroids?" in SCIENCE AND SPORTING PERFORMANCE: MANAGEMENT OR MANIPULATION?, edited by B. Davies and G. Thomas. Oxford, 1982, pp.121-136.

International Athletic Foundation. SAVE THE FUTURE SAVE YOURSELF. AN ANTI-DOPING CAMPAIGN ON BEHALF OF YOUNG ATHLETES. Monte Carlo: The Foundation, 1988. 23pp.

Johnson, R. E. "Do ergogenic aids really improve performance?" in EXERCISE NUTRITION AND PERFORMANCE: PROCEEDINGS OF THE 5TH BIENNIAL CONFERENCE, edited by P. Russo and G. Gass. Sydney: Cumberland College of Health Sciences, Sports Sciences and Research School, 1985. pp. 160-165.

Keen, C. L. and R. M. Hackman. "Trace Elements in Athletic Performance" in SPORT, HEALTH AND NUTRITION, edited by F. I. Katch. Champaign, Illinois: Human Kinetics, 1986. pp.51-65.

Keenan, E. J. "Anabolic and androgenic steroids" in DRUGS, ATHLETES, AND PHYSICAL PERFORMANCE, edited by J. A. Thomas. New York: Plenum Medical Book Company, 1988. pp.91-103.

Kerr, R., M.D. THE PRACTICAL USE OF ANABOLIC STEROIDS WITH ATHLETES. San Gabriel, California: Robert Kerr Publishing, 1982.
> Dr. Robert Kerr, physician, had been treating athletes with anabolic steroids for many years when he wrote this book to share his experience and expertise. He discussed a number of topics including: laboratory tests; diet and supplements; specific anabolic steroids; human growth hormone; human chorionic gonadotropin; and other drugs related to athletics; their side effects, dosages and costs.

Kohoe, P. RELEVANCE OF ANABOLIC STEROIDS TO MIDDLE DISTANCE RUNNING. Australian Track and Field Coaches Association, Sydney, 1982. pp. 21.

Lamb, D. R. PROLONGED EXERCISE, Indianapolis: Benchmark, 1988.

Lapchick, R. E., and R. Malokoff. ON THE MARK: PUTTING THE STUDENT BACK IN STUDENT-ATHLETE. Lexington, Massachusetts: D. C. Health and Company, 1987. 215 pp.

Latour, M. E. THE EFFECTS OF ANABOLIC STEROIDS ON HDL-C LEVELS IN MALE BODYBUILDERS (dissertation). Eugene, Oregon: Microform Publications, 1987. 2 microfiches. 102 fr.

Llewellyn, G., and G. Poole. THE JOY OF FLEX: A THINKING MAN AND WOMAN'S GUIDE TO BASIC BODYBUILDING, 2nd ed. Ottawa: Carleton Physicial Recreation Centre, 1986. 297pp.
Anabolic steroids discussed on pp.242-247.

Markku, A. EFFECTS OF SELF-ADMINISTERED, HIGH-DOSE TESTOS-TERONE AND ANABOLIC STEROIDS ON SERUM HORMONES, LIPIDS, ENZYMES AND ON SPERMATOGENESIS IN POWER ATHLETES, Jyvaskyla, Finland: The University, 1985. 75 pp.

Mitchell, B. J. SERUM TESTOSTERONE AND ESTRADIOL-17 BETA LEVELS RELATIVE TO THE PERFORMANCE CAPABILITIES OF NONATHLETIC FEMALES (dissertation). Eugene, Oregon: Microform Publications, 1983. 1 microfiche.

Mohun, J. DRUGS, STEROIDS AND SPORTS. New York: Watts, 1988. 62 pp.
This book explains how drugs entered sports, names drugs used, and describes the desired and harmful effect for young readers in junior high. A final chapter, "winning without drugs," offers practical advice to young athletes who wish to be competitive without potentially endangering themselves.

Munch, L. R. DRUGS AND THE ATHLETE. Haycock, C. E. 1980, pp. 351-361.
Three pages are devoted to a brief general introduction to anabolic steroids and discussion of adverse side effects, mainly the link between steroids and liver cancer.

NATIONAL COLLEGIATE ATHLETIC ASSOCIATION. The 1988-1989 NCAA Drug Testing Program. Mission, Kansas: NCAA, 1988. 20 pp.

Novich, N. M. and B. Taylor. TRAINING AND CONDITIONING OF ATHLETES, 2nd ed. Philadelphia: Lea & Febiger, 1983.

Nuzzo, N. A. and D. P. Waller. "Drug Abuse in Athletes" in DRUGS, ATHLETES AND PHYSICAL PERFORMANCE, edited by J. A. Thomas. New York: Plenum, 1988. pp.141-167.

Puffer, J. C. "Drugs and Doping in Athletics" in SPORTS INJURIES AND ATHLETIC PROBLEMS, edited by Morris B. Mellion. St. Louis: Mosby, 1988. pp.37-48.

Rakel, R. E. CONN'S CURRENT THERAPY. Philadelphia: Saunders, 1989. pp.293, 569-572.

Rippe, J. M. and W. Southmayd. THE SPORTS PERFORMANCE FACTORS. Putman, New York: 1986. 208 pp.
Anabolic steroid use is discussed on pp. 185-186 along with cocaine abuse and blood doping. Most of this book is devoted to conditioning, flexibility, strength training, mental strategies, nutrition and performance.

Rogol, A. D. "Growth Hormone: Physiology, Therapeutic Use, and Potential for Abuse" in EXERCISE AND SPORT SCIENCES REVIEWS 17. Baltimore: Williams and Wilkins, 1989. pp.353-377.

Roy, S. USE OF DRUGS IN SPORTS. Bell. G. W. Proceedings of the Profession-al Preparation Conferences: National Athletic Trainers Association, Champaign, Ill. Human Kinetics Publishers, 1982. pp. 116-124.

Written for athletic trainers to recognize indications, dosage, and side effects of medications used in training room setting. Corticosteroids and anabolic steroids each have about a page of discussion along with other drugs.

Schade, D. S. "Stress hormone response to exercise" in SPORTS MEDICINE; FITNESS, TRAINING, INJURIES, edited by Otto Appenzeller. Baltimore; Urban and Schwarzenberg. 1988. pp. 181-187.

SPORTS AND DRUG ABUSE, HEARING BEFORE THE SUBCOMMITTEE ON ALCOHOLISM AND DRUG ABUSE OF THE COMMITTEE ON LABOR AND HUMAN RESOURCES, UNITED STATES SENATE, NINETY-EIGHT CONGRESS, SECOND SESSION, September 25, 1984. Washington, D. C.: Senate Committee on Labor and Human Resources, 1985. 67 pp.

STEROIDS: SHORTCUT TO MAKE-BELIEVE MUSCLES. Niles, Illinois: United Learning, 1988. Color videotape. 32 min. $125.
This is a simply and clearly done videotape produced to educate the general population to the dangers of anabolic steroids. Experts offer advice on potential harmful effects and a coach offers a training program based on scientific principles.

Stone, M. H. "Androgens and growth hormone" in SPORTS MEDICINE HAND-BOOK, edited by K. Faeth. Colorado: The United States Weightlifting Federation, 1986. pp.65-68.

Strauss, R. H. "Anabolic steroid use by young athletes" in COMMON PROB-LEMS IN PEDIATRIC SPORTS MEDICINE, edited by N. J. Smith. Chicago: Year Book Medical Publishers, 1989. pp 131-135.

Taylor, W. N. ANABOLIC STEROIDS AND THE ATHLETE. McFarland, Jefferson, N. C.: 1982. 116 pp.
Introduces the continuing controversy; gives description of compounds, anabolic to androgenic ratio; discusses basic principles in protein synthe-sis; reviews studies with male subjects; and provides basic theories behind regimes with oral and injectable preparations, HGH, detection, liver diseases, etc.

—. HORMONAL MANIPULATION: A NEW ERA OF MONSTROUS ATHLETES. Jefferson: McFarland and Company, 1985. 44 pp.

Ungerleider. S. DRUGS IN SPORTS: AN OVERVIEW. Eugene, Oregon: Integrated Research Services, 1986. 17 pp.

United States. House. CONTROLLED SUBSTANCES ACT (ANABOLIC STEROIDS) HEARING. Committee on the Judiciary. Subcommittee on Crime. Legislation to amend the controlled substances act. H. R. 3216. July 27, 1988. 1989. 105 pp.

Wadler, G. I. DRUGS AND THE ATHLETE. Philadelphia: F. A. Davis, 1989. 353 pp.
This is an authoritative book covering every aspect of legal and illegal drugs and athletes. Anabolic steroids are included along with cocaine, blood doping, diuretics, etc.; historical summaries physiology, and adverse effects also included. Drug testing and legal considerations are discussed; Extensive bibliographics provided after each chapter; and

appendixes are full of drug policies and position statements by major sport organizations.

Weider, J. and B. Reynolds. COMPETITIVE BODYBUILDING. Chicago: Comtemporary Books, 1984. 172 pp.

Weiner, B. DRUG ABUSE IN SPORTS: ANNOTATED BIBLIOGRAPHY. Brooklyn: Compu-Bibs, 1985.

Williams, M. H. BEYOND TRAINING: HOW ATHLETES ENHANCE PERFORM-ANCE LEGALLY AND ILLEGALLY. Champaign: Human Kinetics, 1989.
This is a comprehensive, factual, clearly presented reference on ergo-genic aids in sports; it provides background on why and how athletes use ergogenic aids. Nutrition aids, pharmacologic aids, psychological strate-gies and mechanical aids are described.

—, editor. ERGOGENIC AIDS IN SPORT. Champaign: Human Kinetics, 1983.

Wilmore, J. H. "Physiological effects of strength training and various strength training devices" in PROFESSIONAL PREPARATION IN ATHLETIC TRAINING: PROCEEDINGS OF THE PROFESSIONAL PREPARATION CONFERENCES; NATIONAL ATHLETIC TRAINERS ASSOCIATION. Arizona: The National Athletic Trainers Association, 1982. p. 8.

Wong, G. M. ESSENTIALS OF AMATEUR SPORTS LAW. Dover, Massachusetts: Auburn House, 1988. pp.597-631.
This reference book has thorough coverage of drug testing in amateur athletics, discussing intercollegiate, interscholastic and Olympic compe-tition.

Woodland, L. "The Builders" in DOPE: THE USE OF DRUGS IN SPORT. London: Newton Abbot, 1980. pp.53-82.
This chapter provides a readable history, stories about world and Olympic athletes, records held and their anabolic steroid use.

Wright, J. E. ANABOLIC STEROIDS AND SPORTS, vol. II. Natick: Sports Science Consultants, 1982.
These two volumes are by an exercise scientist who evaluated animal studies available in 1977 and shared personal observations of the use and effects of drugs in athletes; many selected references.

—. "Anabolic-androgenic steroids" in ATHLETES AT RISK: DRUGS AND SPORT, edited by R. Tricker and D. L. Cook. Dubuque, Iowa: W. C. Brown, 1990. pp.53-72.

Periodical Literature

Overview

Anabolic-androgenic steroids, by J. E. Kristensen. SCIENTIFIC METHODICAL BULLETIN 2:13-15, 1979

Anabolic steroid use among athletes and the future, by H. E. Lzumi. ATHLETIC TRAINING 25(1): 58+, Spring 1990
> This is a fine overview article that discusses supply, dosage, techniques, effects, and approaches to solve the problem of anabolic steroid use.

Anabolic steroids and athletics, by J. E. Wright. EXERCISE AND SPORT SCIENCES REVIEWS 8:149-202, 1980
> A very thorough overview with extensive references is provided, including the development of anabolic steroids, nature of the protein anabolic response, mechanism of action, training studies and health risks.

Anabolic steroids and Norwegian weightlifters, by S. Solberg. BRITISH JOURNAL OF SPORTS MEDICINE 16(3):169-171, September 1982

Anabolic steroids and sport, by R. Rigby. AUSTRALIAN WEIGHTLIFTERS 4-6, November 1981

Anabolic steroids and strength and power related athletic events, by D. R. Lamb. JOURNAL OF PHYSICAL EDUCATION AND RECREATION 51(2):58-59, February 1980
> Lamb provides a brief overview and pleas for massive educational campaign to dissuade youth from abusive anabolic steroids.

Anabolic steroids are fool's gold, by A. J. Ryan. FEDERATION OF AMERICAN SOCIETIES FOR EXPERIMENTAL BIOLOGY, FEDERATION PROCEEDINGS 40(12):2682-2688, October 1981
> After an excellent historical introduction to the use of anabolic steroids and high-protein diets in strength sports, Ryan reviews results of published studies on the effectiveness of anabolic steroids, discusses testing, and provides an extensive bibliography of references published before 1980 when this paper was presented at a symposium, DRUG USE IN ATHLETICS, in Anaheim, California.

Anabolic steroids breakfast of champions?, by R. Lopez. FAHPER JOURNAL
17(2):18-21, May 1979
> This is an excellent overview article with 43 references published before
> 1979. The author discusses who uses anabolic steroids, side effects,
> possible benefits, research studies on anabolic steroids, protein supple-
> ments, and the coach's responsibility for the health and well being of
> athletes.

Anabolic steroids in sports: a biophysical evaluation, by J. P. O'Shea. CANADIAN
ATHLETIC THERAPISTS ASSOCIATION JOURNAL 6(1):5-12, March 1979

Anabolic steroids: a review of the literature, by H. A. Haupt, et al. AMERICAN
JOURNAL OF SPORTS MEDICINE 12:469-484, 1984.
> This is the most detailed review of medical and scientific literature.

Anabolic steroids: the gremlins of sport, by T. Todd. JOURNAL OF SPORT
HISTORY 14:87-107, Spring 1987.
> This is an excellent historical review of popular and professional literature.

Anabolic steroids use and abuse profile in Canada, by M. Desgagne, et al. CANA-
DIAN PHARMACEUTICAL JOURNAL August 1989, pp. 402-408
> This is an excellent overview article that covers abuse of anabolic steroids
> by recreational body-builders and competitive athletes; human growth
> hormone use, adverse side effects; production, consumption, trade and
> trafficking; chemistry and clinical data; and trade names with usual dosage
> for androgen deficiency.

Anabolics: let your anger rip. Part 1. Anabolic-androgenic steroids in bodybuilding and sport, by J. E. Wright. MUSCLE AND FITNESS 42(11):68-71+,
November 1981

Anabolics: let your anger rip. Part 2. Properties and development of androgens
and anabolic steroids, by J. E. Wright. MUSCLE AND FITNESS 42I12):50-
51+, December 1981

Athletic polydrug abuse phenomenon, by J. A. Hill, et al. AMERICAN JOURNAL
OF SPORTS MEDICINE 11(4):269-271, July/August 1983
> A case report of an injured power weight lifter is presented to demon-
> strate the high doses of anabolic steroids that athletes use without
> medical supervision and despite knowledge of serious side effects.

Coercive power of drugs in sports, by T. H. Murray. HASTINGS CENTER RE-
PORT 13(4):24-30, August 1983
> This extensive historical overview of the non medical use of drugs to
> enhance performance discusses at length the ethical dilemma of using
> drugs to gain that competitive edge.

Chemical bodybuilding, by J. Everson. MUSCLE DIGEST 6(2):32-35+, March
1982

Curbing the use of steroids in American football, by K. Kontor. NATIONAL
STRENGTH AND CONDITIONING ASSOCIATION JOURNAL 10(3):72,
June/July 1988
> This is an editorial recommending random and unannounced testing with
> severe penalties for offenders as well as changing the rules to emphasize
> speed and endurance over strength, size and explosive power. The
> author suggests that the game would be more like Canadian football or

even rugby and training demands would change and thus lessen the benefit of taking steroids.

Drugs: amphetamines and anabolic steroids, and athletic performance, by R. Neil. SPORTS SCIENCE PERIODICAL ON RESEARCH AND TECHNOLOGY IN SPORT (2):1-3, 1979

Drugs and exercise, by D. P. Lowenthal. SPORTSMEDICINE DIGEST 4(11):1-3, November 1982

Drugs and sport, by M. F. Stuck. ARENA REVIEW 12(1):1+, May 1988
This whole issue is devoted to drugs and sports and includes articles on drug use among professional hockey players, a survey of selected N.A.I.A. colleges in Kansas which includes information on anabolic steroids use, and guidelines for a drug control program.

Drugs in sport: the extent of the problem, toxic effects, and control, by C. I. Arblaster, et al. AUSTRALIAN FAMILY PHYSICIAN 10(3):145-146+, March 1981
This article discusses both the desired and unwanted effects from the use of amphetamines and anabolic steroids and then explains dope testing.

Drugs in sports, by H. C. Mofenson, et al. NEW YORK STATE JOURNAL OF MEDICINE 80(1):57-60, January 1980
Written for medical personnel, coaches and trainers who need information about drug use and misuse in sport, authors cover stimulants, analgesics, anti-latal anesthetics, and sedative tranquilizers.

Effects of anabolic steroids on strength development and performance, by P. J. Stackpole. NATIONAL STRENGTH COACHES ASSOCIATION JOURNAL 2(2):30-33, March/April 1980

Ergogenic aids in swimming, by E. R. Burke. SWIMMING WORLD AND JUNIOR SWIMMER 22(1):71-74, January 1981

Facts about anabolic steroids, by E. Darden. ATHLETIC JOURNAL 63:100-101, March 1983
This is a succinct review of the history of steroid use, research studies, discussion of the placebo effect and side effects.

Getting tough on anabolic steroids: can we win the battle?, by J. A. Shroyer. PHYSICIAN AND SPORTSMEDICINE 18(2):106-110, February 1990

Great steroid myth, by G. Shepard. SCHOLASTIC COACH 58:60-62, March 1989
Dr. Greg Shepard, president of Bigger Faster Stronger, which conducts clinics for high school athletes, has written an article in question and answer format to clarify what happens when an athlete uses steroids; also provides examples of successful athletes who do not use steroids.

Illegal steroid use among fifty weightlifters, by J. R. Fuller, et al. SOCIOLOGY AND SOCIAL RESEARCH 73(1):19-21, October 1988.
This article provides some insights into why weightlifters use illegal steroids with some surprising results about enhanced sexual drive and pleasure, lack of knowledge of potential consequences, and dissimilarity with recreational drug users.

Ingestion, injection, and the competitive edge, by D. R. Lamb. NATIONAL ASSO-
CIATION FOR PHYSICAL EDUCATION IN HIGHER EDUCATION PROCEED-
INGS 47-55, 1979

Making of a champion: chemistry or coaching, by A. Pipe. SPORTS (2):1-6, De-
cember 1983
This same paper was published in TRACK AND FIELD QUARTERLY
REVIEW, VOLUME 88, 1988, but originally presented at the Fifth Annual
National Coaches' Seminar held October 20-23, 1983 at Mont Ste. Marie,
Quebec. This is an editorial and commentary on drugs and sports with
some helpful explanations and definitions.

National Institute on Drug Abuse may join in anabolic steroid research by V. S.
Cowart. JAMA 261:1855-1856, April 7, 1989
This report summarizes issues raised by experts at the NIDA meeting
about the use of anabolic steroids: psychiatric effects, drug testing, and
the need for funding of research on short and long term effects.

Nutrition: anabolic steroids—where we stand today, by A. Grandjean. NATIONAL
STRENGTH AND CONDITIONING ASSOCIATION JOURNAL 3(6):58-59+,
December 1981/January 1982

Pervasive anabolic steroid use among health club athletes, by W. N. Taylor, et al.
ANNALS OF SPORTS MEDICINE 3:155-159, 1987.

Simple facts about anabolic steroids, by R. Rigby. MODERN ATHLETE AND
COACH 19(4):19-20, October 1981

Steroids muscle in on the world of bodybuilding. JOURNAL OF SPORTS MEDI-
CINE AND PHYSICAL FITNESS 19(2):228, June 1979

Steroids . . . pumping trouble. IMPACT: NEWSLETTER OF CHEMICAL HEALTH
IN WOMEN 4(3), Fall 1988
This article gives definitions, provides common brand names, reports
briefly on results of national survey of health club athletes, and summarizes health risks.

Steroids: their pharmacological properties, by R. A. Palermo. TRACK TECH-
NIQUE 82:2609-2610, Winter 1981

Use and abuse of drugs in sport, by A. H. Beckett. JOURNAL OF BIOSOCIAL
SCIENCE SUPPLEMENT 7:163-170, 1981
Beckett comments on the increasing misuse of drugs in sport, attempts
to test for and control drugs misused, devices used to evade detection,
and efforts by different countries to curtail the problem. Author strongly
urges international cooperation in testing efforts and disqualifications.

Use of anabolic steroids poses major risk to athletes, by C. S. Blyth, et al. NA-
TIONAL COLLEGIATE ATHLETIC ASSOCIATION NEWS 18(13):3, Septem-
ber 15, 1981

Use and abuse of steroids: the American College of Sports Medicine issues a
statement condemning the burgeoning use of anabolic-androgenic steroids
by competitive athletes, by A. Tanny. MUSCLE AND FITNESS 42(9):58-59+,
September 1981

Use of anabolic steroids by elite athletes studies, by M. Moore. PHYSICIAN AND
SPORTSMEDICINE 9(7):22, July 1981

This is a brief report on a study of 12 national level athletes who admitted two years of anabolic steroid use. Users were compared to 8 athletes who had never taken steroids and 15 untrained men. Muscle biopsies showed that "the size of the muscle fibers was unrelated to the individual's size, amount of training, or use of anabolic steroids."

Use of anabolic steroids by national level athletes, by D. Pearson, et al. NATIONAL STRENGTH COACHES ASSOCIATION JOURNAL 3(2):16-18, April/May 1981

Use of anabolic steroids in athletics, by M. Stone, et al. JOURNAL OF DRUG ISSUES 10(3):351-359, Summer 1980
This is a synopsis of research findings from mostly animal and some human studies, but conclusions are unclear. Authors summarize that anabolic steroids probably increase performance in some athletes due to the effect on the central nervous system and not protein anabolism.

Use of ergogenic aids, by J. F. Cirrito. TRACK TECHNIQUE 77:2444-2446, Fall 1979

General

After breakfast failed, by R. Baker. NEW YORK TIMES January 7, 1987, p. 27
>After giving his opinions on the topic of drugs in sports, the author explains and defines doping, drug therapy and drug abuse in sports including the use of steroids.

All you ever wanted to know about steroids, by R. Metz. MUSCULAR DEVELOPMENT 16(3):12-13+, 1979

Anabolic actions, by R. Sullivan, et al. SPORTS ILLUSTRATED 64:13, April 21, 1986

Anabolic drug use examined by NSCA. TEXAS COACH February 1986, p. 43

Anabolic steroids: pumping trouble, by A. Hecht. FDA CONSUMER 18(4):12-15, September 1984

Anabolic steroids: the power and the glory?, by R. E. Ferner, et al. BRITISH MEDICAL JOURNAL 297(6653):877-87, October 8, 1988

Anabolic steroids: what are the consequences?, by C. Jastremski. SWIMMING WORLD AND JUNIOR SWIMMER 20(1):53, January 1979

Anabolic stimulus, by M. Colgan. MUSCLE AND FITNESS July 1988, p.27+

Athletes and steroids: the bad bargain, by V. S. Cowart. SATURDAY EVENING POST 259:56-59, April 1987
>This is an excellent overview of the topic including when steroid use was first introduced in the U.S., definitions and differences between corticosteroids and anabolic steroids, how testing is done, side effects, and pressure to use as described by one former olympic contender and physician.

Athletes doubt drug use will diminish , by F. Litsky. NEW YORK TIMES September 28, 1988, p.D32

Bosworth barred for steroid use (Brian Bosworth). NEW YORK TIMES December 26, 1986, p.D7

Breakfast of champions, by L. Lasagna. THE SCIENCES 24:61-62, March/April 1984
>Reports that Jeff Michels, weightlifter, and other athletes were disqualified at the Pan American Games when urinalysis tests showed abnormally

high levels of testosterone; many others left before their events and urine tests; also reviews side effects

Case against steroids. Doctors find no convincing evidence that the drug improves an athlete's performance - but ample proof that they are dangerous. by N. Angier. DISCOVER 98-101, November 1983
This is an excellent overview of the history of both natural and synthetic steroids, how they are thought to work on muscle tissue, and the unwelcome side effects on men and women.

Character, not chemistry must take the gold, by G. F. Will. LOS ANGELES TIMES September 29, 1988, Section II, p. 7

Chemistry of competition: drugs and the Olympic athlete by L. Thompson. WASHINGTON POST September 13, 1988, p.WH12
A related article on ethical aspects of athletes and drugs is included.

Colleges learn that testing athletes for steroids won't be easy or cheap, by P. Monaghan. CHRONICLE OF HIGHER EDUCATION 30:27-28, May 8, 1985
This article briefly summarizes test experts' warnings about the lack of quality labs and medical personnel as well as leading opinions on such issues as making anabolic steroids controlled substances and/or random unannounced testing of athletes.

Combating chemical warfare: ergogenic aids in sports, by C. E. Percy. SPORTS MEDICINE DIGEST 4:4-5, November 1982
This articles provides a very general introduction to ergogenic aids in sports grouped into five categories: physiological, physical, psychological, nutritional and chemical.

Curbing the use of steroids in American football , by K. Kontor. NATIONAL STRENGTH AND CONDITIONING ASSOCIATION JOURNAL 10(3): 72, June/July 1988

Dangerous edge, by J. C. Horn. PSYCHOLOGY TODAY 17:68, November 1983

Description of steroids (brief definition of difference between anabolic and cortical steroids). NEW YORK TIMES November 17, 1988, p.B12

Dissident attacks Soviet sports system (Yuri Vlasov accuses Soviets of disregarding use of steroids by athletes), by F.Barringer. NEW YORK TIMES October 2, 1988, p. 27

Doping, by C. A. Mireles. TEXAS COACH 28(9): 18-19, May 1985

Doping for the competitive edge (sports). WORLD PRESS REVIEW 36:59, June 1989

Drug abuse: steroids, stimulants a problem, by D. Middleton. RUGBY LEAGUE WEEK 20(27):3, August 23, 1989

Drugs at the Olympics. WASHINGTON POST September 29, 1988, p.A20

Epidemic in sports: steroids, by D. Anderson. NEW YORK TIMES 1(1):56, July 10, 1988

Ergogenic aids: no substitute for proper training, by E. Burke. VELO-NEWS 8(16):3, October 1979

Ergogenic aids, by D. Graetzer. HANDBALL 38:26-27, October 1988

Experts say steroids often benefit, pose health risks, by K. McDonald. CHRONI-CLE OF HIGHER EDUCATION 30:27-29, May 8, 1985
  This short article summarizes the health risks attributed to steroids' use.

Federal agency to probe anabolic steroids abuse. PHYSICIAN AND SPORTS-MEDICINE 17(7):16-17, July 1989
  The National Institute on Drug Abuse (NIDA) plans a major investigation of steroid abuse; key issue being dependency.

First for Canada: Toronto athlete banned from competition, by P. Gains. ATH-LETICS 9-11, May 1982

For a drug-free sport, by J. Kuc. MUSCLE AND FITNES 45(2):89+, February 1984

Former Husker fesses up , by A. Keteyian. SPORTS ILLUSTRATED 66:24, January 5, 1987
  Dean Steinkuhler admits former use of steroids at Nebraska and with Oilers.

Game of cat and mouse: there's a new olympic event pitting athletes against drug busters. U.S. NEWS AND WORLD REPORT 105:38, October 10, 1988

Griffith Joyner sets mark; 2nd gold for Joyner-Kersee; Hungarian weightlifter fails drug test (Andor Szanyi), by G. Solomon, et al. WASHINGTON POST September 29, 1988, p.A1

Guru who spreads the gospel of steroids (Dan Duchaine), by P. Alfano, et al. NEW YORK TIMES November 19, 1988, p.1

High cost of steroids, by H. Quinn. MACLEAN'S 101:45, September 26, 1988
  Athlete's use of steroids is discussed.

How certain drugs can be used to aid competitors. WEIGHTLIFTERS NEWS-LETTER 110: 17, May 5, 1984

Independent study of anabolic steroids, by B. Taylor. MUSCLE DIGEST 3(4):84-85, July/August 1979

Inside dope, by M. Johns. RUNNER'S WORLD 23:78-80, 82-83, September 1988

I.O.C. may study drug use of weight lifters. NEW YORK TIMES 8(2):52, Decem-ber 4, 1988

Is bigger always better?, by E. Nowalkoski. SPORT TALK 15(4): 4, December 1986

Is it worth the risk? Usage of anabolic steroids for performance edge continues, by E. D. Zimper. WRESTLING USA 21(1):7-8, September 1985

Last words on steroids, by F. C. Hatfield. MUSCLE AND FITNESS 45(2):86-87+, February 1984

Lip service: NFL and steroids testing. SPORTS ILLUSTRATED 71(11):20, September 11, 1989

Look at synthetic steroids, by J. Everson. MUSCLE DIGEST 5(5):68-71, December 1981

Looking for a chemcial edge (steroid use by athletes), by C. Wood. MACLEAN'S 102:40, May 13, 1989

Making of a champion : chemistry or coaching?, by A. Pipe. TRACK AND FIELD QUARTERLY REVIEW 88:4-8, 1988
  This is an editorial and overview that explains and defines doping, drug therapy, and drug abuse techniques besides steroids. Definitions are helpful, but the commentary is not always useful.

Medicine: can't ignore the issue, by W. N. Taylor. MUSCLE AND FITNESS 45(2): 88+, February 1984

Mounting menace of steroids, by C. T. Rowan. READER'S DIGEST February 1988, p. 132+

Mounting drug use afflicts world sports, by N. Amdur. BASKETBALL BULLETIN 63-64, 1979

NCAA weight year-round, random drug testing to halt what many call a growing use of steroids, by C. J. Hartley. CHRONICLE OF HIGHER EDUCATION 35: 35-36, January 11, 1989

New breakfast of champions: a recipe for victory or disaster?, by L. K. Altman. NEW YORK TIMES November 20, 1988, p.1

Olympic images, by H. Quinn. MACLEAN'S 102:33, January 2, 1989

Peril for athletes, by R. Telander. SPORTS ILLUSTRATED 69:114, October 24, 1988

Playing to win and looking good, by B. Berube. CANADIAN PHARMACEUTICAL JOURNAL August 1989, pp. 410+

Pre-Olympic games, now in progress, demand world-class medical teamwork, by V. S. Cowart. JAMA 258(6):741-742, August 14, 1987
  William Grana, M. D. chief physician for the U.S. athletes in the Pan-American games in Indianapolis is interviewed and comments on his one worry of finding a positive drug test in an athlete and the bad publicity that would follow. Sports drug testing is described as well as the groups of banned drugs. Requirements for U. S. Olympic team physicians are also briefly explained.

Researchers establish dangers of steroids , by S. M. Kleiner. NEW YORK TIMES December 28, 1988, p.A14

Roll up to see the bearded ladies (drug use by olympic athletes). ECONOMIST 309: 45, October 1, 1988

Sex hormones and athletes. HEALTH LETTER 23(9):1-2, May 11, 1984

Shocking stain on international athletics, by R. Chelminski. READER'S DIGEST August 1988, p.131
> West German Birgit Dressel's death in 1987 is reported; David Jenkins, British Olympic Silver medalist, pleaded guilty in San Diego to taking part in multi-million dollar a year U.S. drug ring that specialized in anabolic steroids, HGH and HCG . Recommends punishment for abusers, random testing and classification of steroids HGH and HCG as controlled substances.

Steroid data cited and disputed. NEW YORK TIMES (1):29, June 15, 1989

Steroid debate: enhanced vs. natural athletes, by O. Connolly. WASHINGTON POST September 13, 1988, p.WH15

Steroid edge: real or illusion? Experts doubt the effects reported on athletes' muscles, by F. S. Chapman. WASHINGTON POST October 18, 1988, p.8

Steroid generation, by R. Goldman, et al. MUSCLE TRAINING ILLUSTRATED 79:32-33+, October 1979

Steroid predicament (in spite of evidence that anabolic steroids can undermine one's health, the use of these drugs is widespread among athletes, who will risk their physical well-being for the promise of stronger performance), by T. Todd. SPORTS ILLUSTRATED 59(5): 62-66+, August 1, 1983

Steroid scandal, by C. Francis. MACLEAN'S 102(2):36-42, March 13, 1989

Steroid scandal, by D. Burke. MACLEAN'S 102:40, February 20, 1989

Steroids, by L. Woodland. INTERNATIONAL CYCLE SPORT 129:11, February 1979

Steroids: a clinical update, by A. Nayes. MUSCLE AND FITNESS 47(3):48-51+, March 1986

Steroids: demon of death, by B. Goldman. MUSCLE TRAINING 77(27):39-40+, July 1979

Steroids '84. YOUR HEALTH AND FITNESS 6(3):26-27, June/July 1984

Steroids: a problem of huge dimensions (by using anabolic steroids, athletes like Tampa Bay Bucs' Steve Courson are looking for an edge and maybe for trouble), by W. D. Johnson. SPORTS ILLUSTRATED 62(19): 38-42+, May 13, 1985

Steroids: the power drugs, by P. Pfotenhauer. USA TODAY 117:88-90, March 1989
> This is an excellent, readable, general introduction to steroid use, side effects, pressure on athletes to be competitive, increased sports injuries and steroid testing. A glossary of some of the more popular steroids and their desired effects is included. The psychological and physical dependence on steroids is emphasized by the two California sports medicine specialists.

Steroids: the stuff of synthetic supermen?, by M. S. Kreiter. CURRENT HEALTH 14:14-16, December 1987
> This article presents a basic, simple explanation of steroids and their effect on the human body.

Substance abuse and sportsmanship, by S. Ross. CAHPER JOURNAL 55(4):35-38, July/August 1989
> This is an editorial response to a Canadian sports columnist's plea for the removal of anabolic steroids from the banned substances list; Mr. Ross contends that the sports columnist's article and viewpoint "does not enhance sport."

Super athletes made to order: new synthetic hormones give the "win at any cost" philosophy an even deadlier meaning in today's sports, by W. N. Taylor. PSYCHOLOGY TODAY 19(5):62-66, May 1985

Suspension of twenty-one football players from Bowl Games for taking steroids: reviews debate over purpose of drug tests and appropriate penalties, by D. Lederinan. CHRONICLE OF HIGHER EDUCATION 33:34+, January 7, 1987

They shoot, they score: the inside dope on drug use in the locker rooms of the nation, by H. Bruce. QUEST: CANADA'S URBAN MAGAZINE 116:118, November 1981

Update on anabolic steroids, by L. J. Silvester. SCHOLASTIC COACH 48(9):74+, April 1979

Users and losers, by J. Henderson. RUNNER'S WORLD 24:14, March 1989

Using chemistry to get the gold: steroids and hormones are sometimes the building blocks of Olympic glory, by P. Axthelm. NEWSWEEK July 25, 1988, p.62

Victory at any cost: drug pressure growing, by M. Janofsky, et al. NEW YORK TIMES November 21, 1988, p.A 1

Weight lifter used drug (1988 Olympic weight lifting silver medalist Andor Szanyi). NEW YORK TIMES September 29, 1988, p.54

Winking at steroids in sports. NEW YORK TIMES November 22, 1988, p.A14

Ben Johnson

Advisors around Ben, by D. Jenish. MACLEAN'S 101:54-56, October 10, 1988

Agony of victory. CHRISTIAN SCIENCE MONITOR September 29, 1988, p.13

Athletes' steroid use causing deep concern, by L. K. Altman. NEW YORK TIMES September 28, 1988, p.52

Ban on Johnson is a life saver, by G. Vecsey. NEW YORK TIMES. September 28, 1988, p.52
> Ben Johnson's positive drug test for steroid use is seen as an opportunity to increase athletes' awareness of drug's negative effects.

Ben Johnson, world's fastest scapegoat, by N. Fost. NEW YORK TIMES October 20, 1988, p.23

Ben's new challenges: B. Johnson on even of Canadian Inquiry into role of drugs in sport, by C. Wood. MACLEAN'S 101:45, November 21, 1988

Better living through chemistry a fallacy: Ben Johnson lost gold medal when he tested positive for steroids. SPORTING NEWS 206:15, October 10, 1988

Canada examines amateur system, by J. F. Burns. NEW YORK TIMES October 16, 1988, p.25

Coach says Johnson took steroids since 1981; ex-gold medalist was told all top ranked sprinters used drugs: Ben Johnson, by H. H. Denton. WASHINGTON POST 4:1, March 2, 1989

Day of reckoning: Ben Johnson admits he took steroids. MACLEAN'S 102:32, June 26, 1989

Deepening scandal: physician J. Astaphan testifies on steroids used by B. Johnson, by B. Wickens. MACLEAN'S 102:49-50, June 5, 1989

Dirty coach comes clean, by M. Noden. SPORTS ILLUSTRATED 70:22-23, March 13, 1989

Disgraced Canadian sprinter Johnson crosses a grim finish line at home, by H. H. Denton. WASHINGTON POST September 28, 1988, p.A26

Dope and glory: anabolic steroids used by B. Johnson, by P. Thompson. RUNNER'S WORLD 23:47, December 1988

Dope and glory: anabolic steroids used by B. Johnson, by P. Thompson. RUNNER'S WORLD 23:47, December 1988

Doped-up games; athletes have been using anabolic steroids for years, but it took the shocking disqualification of Ben Johnson to get the sports world's attention, by P. Axthelm. NEWSWEEK 112: 54, October 10, 1988

Erasing of Johnson: Ben Johnson is stripped of his world records, by H. Hersch. SPORTS ILLUSTRATED 71(12):17, September 18, 1989

Fallout from Seoul, by N. Underwood. MACLEAN'S 101:58, October 17, 1988

Has - Ben: steroid use by B. Johnson disqualifies him from olympic 100-meter win, by A. Burfoot. RUNNER'S WORLD 23:46, December 1988

House of cards,by S. Ballard. SPORTS ILLUSTRATED 69:21, October 17, 1988 Ben Johnson's teammate Angella Issajenko talks about her use of steroids prior to official Canadian inquiry.

Inquiry reaches its heart: Johnson. NEW YORK TIMES 5:10, March 1, 1989

IOC strips Johnson of gold medal in 100: Canadian tests positive for steroid use, C. Brennan. WASHINGTON POST September 27, 1988, p.A1

Johnson admits lying about steroids: Ben Johnson. NEW YORK TIMES 3:11, June 14, 1989

Johnson loses his gold medal over steroids, B. Dwyre. LOS ANGELES TIMES September 27, 1988, Section I, p.1

Johnson saga in perspective: B. Johnson, by A. Fotheringham. MACLEAN'S 101:64, October 10, 1988

Johnson's coach closes with a plea for reform: steroid use by Canadian athletes; Ben Johnson's coach Charlie Francis. NEW YORK TIMES 1:31, March 11, 1989

Johnson's steroid use costs him gold medals, $. JET 75:48, October 17, 1988

Kamsa Hamnida, Ben Johnson (Seoul Olympics analysis; drug use by athletes), by D. Anderson. NEW YORK TIMES October 3, 1988, p.3

Lawyer says doctor had prescribed steroid use: Ben Johnson, Jamie Astraphan. NEW YORK TIMES 4:28, April 6, 1989

Lessons of the Ben Johnson tragedy, by T. Byfield. READER'S DIGEST 134:35, February 1989

Loser, by W. O. Johnson, et al. SPORTS ILLUSTRATED 69(15) : 20-26, October 3, 1988

Loss being suffered by Canadians may be much greater than a medal, J. F. Burns. NEW YORK TIMES September 28, 1988, p.49

No new penalty for Johnson: International Amateur Athletic Federation to take no further action against runner Ben Johnson. NEW YORK TIMES 5:33, March 3, 1989

Record pusher: Ben Johnson and steroids. US NEW AND WORLD REPORT 106:16, March 13, 1989

Revealing inquiry: testimony of J. Astraphan on runner B. Johnson's steroid use, by M. Noden. SPORTS ILLUSTRATED 70:19, June 5, 1989

Sabotage at Seoul?, by R. Dolphin. MACLEAN'S 102:47, March 20, 1989

Saga behind the shame: for the first time, an insider tells what really happened to Ben Johnson last summer, by J. Brant. RUNNER'S WORLD 24(4):78-80, April 1989
> Jack Scott, top sports therapist, tells the author about working with Ben Johnson the summer of 1988 and that Dr. Jamie Astaphan freely admitted prescribing anabolic steroids.

Say it ain't so Ben, Canadian fans appeal to fallen hero, by J. F. Burns. NEW YORK TIMES October 1, 1988, p.34

Second coming for big Ben . . . and then the gold was gone: Ben Johnson wins olympic 100 meter run, loses medal after positive test for steroids. SPORTING NEWS 206:5, October 3, 1988

Shame of the games; Ben Johnson is stripped of his gold in the Olympics' worst drug scandal. TIME 132:74-77, October 10, 1988

Sprinter cites possibility of confusion on steroids: Angella Issajenko, on Ben Johnson's steroid use. NEW YORK TIMES 3:31, March 17, 1989

Steroid scandal, by B. Levin. MACLEAN'S 101:50-53, October 10, 1988

Steroids didn't give him the edge (letter to the editor), by J. C. Valias. WASHINGTON POST October 15, 1988, p.A26

Steroids tied to runner's doctor, by J. F. Burns. NEW YORK TIMES October 7, 1988

When winning can cost too much, by M. T. Kaufman. NEW YORK TIMES September 29, 1988, p.54

When winning is losing: athlete Ben Johnson use of steroids. LOS ANGELES TIMES 1:4, March 5, 1989

Whistle blower. TIME 133:50, March 13, 1989

Children and Adolescents

Young athletes and bodybuilders are using anabolic steroids and human growth hormone to increase the size and strength of their bodies. Recognizing abuse among junior and senior high school students is especially important because excessive amounts of testosterone and its derivatives in the young adolescent may permanently stunt growth. This section includes articles on the extent of use by and side effects of anabolic steroids on children and adolescents.

Adolescent athlete and ergogenic aids, by P. C. Dyment. JOURNAL OF ADO-
LESCENT HEALTH CARE 8(1):68-73, January 1987
> This special issue on medication and drug use in adolescence discusses adolescents' use of drugs to enhance athletic performance, and reviews the real and alleged ergogenic effects and side effects of several drugs to assist physicians in discussing these drugs during the sports physical examination of adolescents.

Anabolic steroid use in adolescence, by W. V. Moore. JAMA 260:3484-3486,
December 16,1988
> This editorial comments on the findings of the Buckley study of high school males: published in the same issue, and covering such topics as the use of anabolic steroids to initiate delayed puberty and promote growth, psychological effects of anabolic steroids, and prevention of use.

Anabolic steroid use: indications of habituation among adolescents, by C. E.
Yesalis, et al. JOURNAL OF DRUG EDUCATION 19(2):103-116, 1989
> This article identifies characteristics of adolescent male anabolic steroid (AS) users and suggests that AS use has a dependence potential. The AS user was found to differ from the nonuser in self-perceptions of health and strength. Also briefly discussed is the use of injectable AS and associated health problems with reusing or sharing needles such as: AIDS and hepatitis. Authors suggest intervention directed at ninth-graders or younger.

Anabolic steroids and the adolescent athlete, by the American Academy of
Pediatrics Committee on Sports Medicine. PEDIATRICS 83(1):127-128,
January 1989
> This article makes a statement condemning the use of anabolic steroids by athletes and gives reasons for deploring their use.

Anabolic-androgenic steroid abuse by athletes, by G. L. White, et al. PHYSICIAN
ASSISTANT 11:43-57, July 1987
> Excellent, well-referenced review covering history, education and side effects.

Anabolic-androgenic steroid use among 1010 men, by H. G. Pope. PHYSICIAN
AND SPORTSMEDICINE 16(7):75-77+, July 1988
Authors sent questionnaires to male students at three U.S. colleges to
obtain some initial information about the prevalence of anabolic-
androgenic steroid use in the U.S.

Androgenic-anabolic steroids in the high school: the new drug crisis, by K.
Mannie. NATIONAL STRENGTH AND CONDITIONING ASSOCIATION
JOURNAL 10(4):64-65, August/September 1988
This article discusses liver dysfunction, the risk of prostate and testicular
cancers and long term health issues associated with non medical use of
steroids, "black-market " steroids.

Are drugs braking gymnasts' growth. PHYSICIAN AND SPORTSMEDICINE 7(11):
18-20, November 1979
The effect could also be explained by diet and strenuous exercise but
observations of soviet female gymnasts suggest that brake drugs may be
used to delay puberty and their growth.

Death of an athlete: Benji Ramirez took steroids to "get big:" they helped make
him a football starter, they may have killed him, by R. Telander, et al. SPORTS
ILLUSTRATED 70(8):68-72+, February 20, 1989

Drug misuse by adolescent athletes, by P. G. Dyment. PEDIATRIC CLINICS OF
NORTH AMERICA29(6):1363-1368, December 1982

Drug use in sports, by M. C. Wilson, et al. PEDIATRIC NURSING 12:452+,
November/December 1986
A brief review of amphetamine and steroid use in athletes for pediatric
nurse practitioner who sent in question.

Drugs and the adolescent athlete, by P. G. Dyment. PEDIATRIC ANNALS 13(8):
602-604, August 1984

Drugs to enhance athletic performance in the adolescent, by A. D. Rogol.
SEMINARS IN ADOLESCENT MEDICINE 1(4):317-324, December 1985

Estimated prevalence of anabolic steroid use among male high school seniors, by
W. E. Buckley, et al. JAMA 260(23):3441-3445, 1988
This article reports the findings of a study of 12th grade male students in
46 private and public high schools. Questionaires were used to establish
a profile of users. Evidence indicates that drug education should begin
as early as junior high and not just for those who participate in school-
based athletics.

For teens, steroids may be bigger issue than cocaine use, by M.Charlier. WALL
STREET JOURNAL, October 4, 1988, pA22

Gauging steroid use in high school kids, by M. Duda. PHYSICIAN AND SPORTS
MEDICINE 16(8):16-17, August 1988
The best way to control steroid use is to improve efforts to educate athletes, coaches and parents about risks, reports a survey of high school
football coaches in Michigan...Arkansas coaches' perceptions about
steroid use in high school football players at large suburban and rural
schools are also explored.

High school kids: looking better, living worse, by R. H. Strauss. PHYSICIAN AND SPORTSMEDICINE 17(2):35, February 1989
> This article presents a one page editorial summarizing and commenting on Buckley and Yesalis et al. study in JAMA (1988) on use at high school level.

High-school athletes and the use of drugs to enhance sports performance, by D. Krowchuik, et al. AMERICAN JOURNAL OF DISEASES OF CHILDREN 142(4):385-386, 1988
> Survey to determine high school athletes' knowledge of and attitudes toward past use of ergogenic aids.

If youngsters overdose with anabolic steroids, what's the cost anatomically and otherwise?, by V. S. Cowart. JAMA 261:1856-1857, April 7, 1989
> This article reports on a National Institute on Drug Abuse meeting on anabolic steroids; endocrinologists and other researchers express concern that young users are taking larger doses than they need to obtain desired physicial effects and that some will end up shorter than they would have been. Case reports of adverse effects and better animal studies are needed to document adverse effects of steroid use.

Medical concerns for the adolescent athlete, by S. G. Taylor, et al. IOWA MEDICINE 77(9):432-437, September 1987

Of steroids and sports. EMERGENCY MEDICINE 20:190-206, February 15, 1988
> This article provides a good overview of the topic from historical and present perspectives including such subjects as: the most commonly abused anabolic steroids; where athletes obtain steroids; legitimate applications; how they work for athletes; adverse effects, especially on female steroid abusers and how to recognize the steroid abuser.

Perceptions of high school strength coaches regarding steroid use: A pilot study. NATIONAL STRENGTH AND CONDITIONING ASSOCIATION JOURNAL 11:67-70, June/July 1989
> This is a report of preliminary findings of a March 1989 pilot study of American high school strength coaches. Designed to obtain information regarding the coaches' perspectives on steroid use in their own high school, this survey had a poor return rate, but the small sample answered questions such as: "do you believe that when combined with heavy weight training and good nutrition, anabolic steroids will stimulate muscle growth, increase size, strength and speed?" and "where do students buy anabolic steroids?"

Performance enhancing drugs in sport: a different form of drug abuse, by J. R. Fuller, et al. ADOLESCENCE 22(88):969-976, Winter 1987
> This article examines the seriousness and prevalence of performance enhancing drugs and the results of a series of interviews with 50 15 to 40-year-old steroid users to determine their attitudes.

Recognizing anabolic steroid abuse, by J. A. Lomardo. PATIENT CARE, August 15, 1985, p.28+
> This article describes clues to anabolic steroid abuse so that physicians can recognize young patients who might be abusing steroids. A chart lists different steroids and acceptable dosages for anabolic effect. Suggestions are offered for monitoring the patient who continues to use steroids.

Scary mix of kids and steroids. US NEWS AND WORLD REPORT 105:13-14, December 26,1988-January 2, 1989

Serum testosterone response to training in adolescent runners, by T. W. Rowland. AMERICAN JOURNAL OF DISEASES OF CHILDREN 141(8):881-883, 1987

Shortcut to the Rambo look, by A. Toufexis. TIME 133:78, January 30, 1989

Spreading use of steroids by young athletes alarms sports medicine specialists, by J. E. Brody. NEW YORK TIMES , February 18, 1988, p.14

Steroids and teens: what parents should know now, by P. Gadsby. GOOD HOUSEKEEPING 205:269, September 1987

Steroids and the young, by C. Neff. SPORTS ILLUSTRATED 69:21, December 26, 1988

Steroids built Mike Keys up; then they tore his down, by M. Brower. PEOPLE WEEKLY 31:107-108, March 20, 1989

Steroids: not just for athletes anymore. PHYSICIAN AND SPORTSMEDICINE 14(6):48, June 1986

Teen steroid use: it's all unsupervised and it's all dangerous, by T. Deters. MUSCLE AND FITNESS 49(5):74-75+, May 1988

Testosterone: what happens when you take it, by D. Prokop. MUSCLE AND FITNESS 47(7):120-122+, July 1986

Trickle-down challenges, by R. Berg. ATHLETIC BUSINESS 13(10):37-39, October 1989
    Increases in steroid use among young athletes is reported as one of the major concerns of athletic directors.

Why children use steroids. NEW YORK TIMES. December 4, 1988, p. S12, sec.1

Young athletes, drinking and drugs: in search of a cure. ATHLETIC BUSINESS 9(9):14+, September 1985
    The problem explored here is drug use among high-school-age youth, and there is no simple solution, say drug-abuse experts. Regardless, there are plenty of people trying to find one.

Education and Counseling

This section lists articles on drug education, advice to coaches, drug counseling, etc., for the purpose of prevention of steroid abuse and encouraging abusers to get into drug rehabilitation programs.

Anabolic steroid enforcement and education actions, by S. L. Nightingale. JAMA 259:178, January 8, 1988
> This is a brief report of the FDA's enforcement efforts to combat anabolic steroid misuse by arresting black market dealers and joint education efforts with the US Department of Education, health and professional societies, the media, etc. to increase public awareness of steroid misuse.

Anabolic steroids: health facts for coaches and athletes, by S. Hannam, et al. SPORTS: SCIENCE PERIODICAL ON RESEARCH AND TECHNOLOGY IN SPORT 1:1-5, September 1987

Baseball: too much scoring. THE ECONOMIST 295:30, June 8, 1985

Basics of a student athlete assistance program, by R. Durall. ATHLETIC DIRECTOR AND COACH 5(3):10-11, March 1987

Bridging the gap: practical application: a realistic approach for strength and conditioning coaches to deal with steroids, by M. Clark. NATIONAL STRENGTH AND CONDITIONING ASSOCIATION JOURNAL 10(2):28-30, April/May 1988.
> The author reviews the more serious side effects and suggests a factual and unbiased education of athletes who know surprisely little about steroids. Author also emphasizes proper diet including supplements along with training to enhance performance.

Coaching strategies for dealing with chemical use. COACHING WOMEN'S BASKETBALL 1(5): 28-29, May/June 1988

Distinction between drug use and abuse, by A. Perry. ATHLETIC TRAINING 20(2):114-116, Summer 1985
> The author outlines major problems associated with steroid use such as liver toxicity and dysfunction, hypertension, undesirable lipoprotein fractions, increased coronary risk, reduced glucose tolerance, gynecomastia, azoospermia and testicular atrophy. On balance, the disadvantages far outweigh the advantages. Potential users are urged to educate themselves about these products and remain under a physician's care. The author also advises coaches on what changes in behavior and/or appearance to look for, so that potential medical problems can be prevented in time.

Drugs and sport, by M. F. Stuck. ARENA REVIEW 12(1):1+, May 1988

Education as a means against doping, by R. O. Voy. FIEP BULLETIN 57:7-13,
1987
Despite the title, this article is mostly about drug testing, which the
author feels can be used as an educational tool against substance abuse
in sport.

Guidelines for a drug control program, by D. C. Pizarro, et al. ARENA REVIEW
12:52-63, May 1988
Objectives of a drug contol program include: justification; individuals to
be tested; substances for which to test; cost of drug testing; frequency
and urine sample collection.

Handling the drug-abusing colleague, by H. Ostro. SCHOLASTIC COACH 57(6):
4+, January 1988

Holtz: steroids won't replace hard work. DRUG FREE ATHLETES 1(1):1, September 1989
This is the front page article of a news letter devoted to fighting against
drugs in sports. Lon Holtz, Notre Dame head football coach, says that
they would not recruit anyone who has used steroids. He also states that
it is easier to explain the negative effects of alcohol and other drugs than
to explain the dangers of steroid use.

Incidence of anabolic steroid use among competitive bodybuilders, by R. Tricker,
et al. JOURNAL OF DRUG EDUCATION 19(4):313-325, 1989
Results of this study of bodybuilders in Kansas and Missouri indicated
that more than half of male bodybuilders compared to 10% of female
competitors used steroids on a regular basis. Bodybuilders felt these
drugs were important for winning and that significant gains in muscle
strength and mass could be achieved by including anabolic steroids as
part of training despite side effects. Authors suggest specific ways to
educate bodybuilders about steroid abuse such as encouraging greater
support from successful nonusers.

Peer counseling pros and cons: beware the "con," by H. Ostro. SCHOLASTIC
COACH 56(9):4+, April 1987
Peer counseling is effective for many issues, but drug abusers are "con"
artists. Peer counselors need constant supervision and special training.
Drug addicts should be removed from school to rehabilitation program.

Performance enhancement in sport. SPORTS MEDICINE:1-6+, January 1989

Physician-competitor's advice to colleagues: steroid users respond to education,
rehabilitation, by V. Cowart. JAMA 257(4):427-428, January 23-30, 1987
Craig Brigham, M. D., and world-class athlete discusses the powerful
placebo effect of anabolic steroids but questions the reported dangers of
steroid use . . . "they may not be any more harmful than oral contraceptives."

Preadolescent strength training, by T. K. Smith. JOURNAL OF PHYSICAL
EDUCATION-RECREATION AND DANCE 55(1):43-44+, January 1984
Physical educators must teach preadolescents about safe and realistic
strength-training methods commensurate with their needs and physical
capabilities. The risk of injuries can be reduced by setting prudent goals,

using equipment tailored to the age level, and educating students about their unique growth state.

Preventing steroid abuse in youth: the health educator's role, by G. L. White, et al. HEALTH EDUCATION 18(4):32-35, August/September 1987
    This article provides a good overview of the growing body of evidence that anabolic-androgenic steroids do NOT increase athletic performance.

Recruit coaches and athletes to help battle drugs, by N. B. Woolf. AMERICAN SCHOOL BOARD JOURNAL 173(2):36, February 1986
    A successful drug and alcohol prevention program developed at Forest Hills School District (Ohio) is described. The program uses athletic coaches to recruit student athletes to support the antidrug program and to bring peer pressure to bear in discouraging drug and alcohol use by their teammates and other students.

Substance abuse policies and guidelines in amateur and professional athletics, by J. C. Wagner. AMERICAN JOURNAL OF HOSPITAL PHARMACY 44(2): 305-310, February 1987
    This article summarizes amateur and professional drug testing policies and guidelines and encourages pharmacists to get involved in drug information and educational services.

Temple's model drug-education program includes tests but emphasizes coun- seling, by C. S. Farrell. CHRONICLE OF HIGHER EDUCATION 33(24): 35-36, February 25, 1987

Theroretical explanation of why athletes choose to use steroids, and the role of the coach in influencing behavior, by G. English. NATIONAL STRENGTH AND CONDITIONING ASSOCIATION JOURNAL 9(4):53-56, August/ September 1987

University of Minnesota's antisteroids campaign aims to tell young athletes why "steroids are big trouble", by E. K. Meintz. AMERICAN SCHOOL AND UNIVERSITY 61:42+, October 1988
    This article briefly describes the U of Minnesota men's Athletic Depart- ment's anti steroid campaign designed to stimulate public awareness through TV and radio announcements and posters. After a summary of serious risks involved with steroid use, the director of the campaign talks about cost and availability of steroids through black market dealers. Sample posters are reproduced and an address provided for further information.

What to say to your athletes about steroids: the long term side effects of steroids are unclear, but coaches and administrators are in a position to combat their use among athletes if they learn to recognize signs of abuse, by R. L. Chambers, et al. ATHLETIC BUSINESS 12(9):54-57, September 1988

HGH and Somatotropin

The extent of human growth hormone (HGH) abuse is unknown partly because it cannot be detected in urine testing at this time. This section includes articles on the potential dangers of growth hormone abuse: acromegaly, stunted growth, shortened life span due to heart disease, and other problems. Several authors recommend that the FDA classify synthetic growth hormone as a controlled substance and not a general prescription drug.

Athletic acromegaly, by W. N. Taylor. POWERLIFTING USA 9(6):20, January 1986

Body composition response to exogenous GH during training in highly conditioned adults, by D. Crist, et al. JOURNAL OF APPLIED PHYSIOLOGY 65(2): 579-584, August 1988
    The effects of chronic alternate-day treatment with supraphysiological doses of biosynthetic methionyl-human GH (met-HGH) on fat-free weight (FFW), percent body fat (% fat), and FFW/FW (fat weight) were investigated in a double-blind, placebo-controlled study with eight well trained young adults.

Breakfast of bigfoot: that's HGH, watch out for it, by F. C. Hatfield. MUSCLE AND FITNESS 48(9):60-61+, September 1987

Drug abuse in athletes: anabolic steroids and human growth hormone, by the Council on Scientific Affairs, American Medical Association. JAMA 259(11): 1703-1705, March 18, 1988
    This article provides an introduction to the problem of misuse of anabolic steroids and growth hormone.

Drugs in sports: human growth hormone used by athletes. VOGUE 177:172, August 1987

Effects of acute physical exercise on blood serum cholesterol, triglycerides, human growth hormone (H.G.H.) and free thryroxine (T4) in men over fifty years of age, by G. Metivier, et al. JOURNAL OF SPORTS MEDICINE AND PHYSICAL FITNESS 28(1):7-10, March 1988

Endocrine roulette, by J. Krakauer. ULTRASPORT 1(5):22-26+, September/ October 1984
    This column focuses on steroids and growth hormones in an attempt to examine how athletes of all types, at all levels, attempt to alter their physiologies to gain a competitive edge.

Gigantic athletes: the dilemma of human growth hormone, by W. N. Taylor. FUTURIST19(4):8-12, 1985

This is a condensed version of the author's book, *Hormonal Manipulation*; author briefly discusses selective gigantism and the "golden girl" scenario as well as controlling synthetic human growth hormone.

Growth hormone, by S. P. Haynes. AUSTRALIAN JOURNAL OF SCIENCE AND MEDICINE IN SPORT 18(1):3-10, March 1986
Growth hormone is now used in sport in an attempt to enhance athletic performance, a situation that may be aggravated by the availability of synthetic growth hormone produced by recombinant DNA techniques.

Growth hormone and athletes, by J. G. Macintyre. SPORTS MEDICINE 4(2):129-142, March/April 1987
This is an excellent, well-referenced overview of the topic; discusses what growth hormone is, its effect on growth, muscle, disorders related to abnormal levels, potential uses and problems.

Growth hormone releasers: what makes you get bigger, by T. Deters, et al. MUSCLE AND FITNESS 47(12):52-53+, December 1986

Growth hormone responses during intermittent weight lifting exercise in men, by W. P. Vanhelder, et al. EUROPEAN JOURNAL OF APPLIED PHYSIOLOGY 53(1):31-34, 1984

Growth hormone: preventing its abuse in sports, by W. N. Taylor. TECHNOLOGY REVIEW 88:14+, October 1985
This article strongly recommends classifying HGH as a controlled substance.

Growth hormone: the latest news about this controversial drug, by J. Nickas. MUSCLE AND FITNESS 47(5):46-47+, May 1986

HGH: the dangerous edge, by L. Allen. WOMEN'S SPORTS AND FITNESS 7(6): 17-18, July 1985
This is a brief, general article about the possible use of growth hormone to increase muscle mass, negative side effects, cost (before synthetic HGH available), inability to test because it occurs naturally in the body, and black market availability of similar "monkey juice" and bovine growth hormone.

Hormonal response during intense exercise preceded by glucose ingestion, by A. Bonen, et al. CANADIAN JOURNAL OF APPLIED SPORTS SCIENCE 5(2):85-80, June 1980

Hormones, exercise and skeletal muscle, by E. A. Richter. SCANDINAVIAN JOURNAL OF SPORTS SCIENCES 8(1):35-41, April 1986

Human growth hormone, by F. C. Hatfield. POWERLIFTING U.S.A. 11(6):18, January 1988

Human growth hormone . . . the herculean horizon, by W. N. Taylor. POWER-LIFTING USA 9(1):28, August 1985

Human growth hormone: promoting its release the natural way, by M. Colgan. MUSCLE AND FITNESS 49(1):74-76+, January 1988

Human growth hormone: use and potential abuse, by M. E. Stachura. HOSPITAL FORMULARY 22(1):48-51+, January 1987

Somatren is a genetically engineered human growth hormone that is commercially available and therapeutically equivalent to somatotropin. This article provides a well-referenced review of its clinical uses as well as potential abuses.

Inhibiting effect of atropine on growth hormone release during exercise, by J. D. Few, et al. EUROPEAN JOURNAL OF APPLIED PHYSIOLOGY 43(3):221-228, 1980

Preventing abuse of human growth hormone, by G. L. White, Jr. PHYSICIAN ASSISTANT 11(7):11-13, July 1987
This editorial warns that HGH may replace steroids as the body-building drug of choice because it cannot be detected in urine.

Regulation of growth hormone during exercise by oxygen demand and availability, by W. P. Vanhelder, et al. EUROPEAN JOURNAL OF APPLIED PHYSIOLOGY AND OCCUPATIONAL PHYSIOLOGY 56(6):628-632, September 1987

Research continues on steroids, growth hormone. FIRST AIDER 54(3):1+, November 1984

Serum prolactin, growth hormone and cortisol in athletes and sedentary subjects after submaximal and exhaustive exercises, by T. Barreca, et al. JOURNAL OF SPORTS MEDICINE AND PHYSICAL FITNESS 28(1):89-92, March 1988
Serum PRL, GH and cortisol values were evaluated in seven athletes and seven sedentary adult subjects after submaximal and exhaustive exercise tests. A significant increase of serum PRL was recorded after the exhaustive exercise in athletes only. Serum GH concentration increase was significant after both exercises in both groups. Serum cortisol concentration underwent an increase after the exhaustive but not after the submaximal exercises in both groups.

Super athletes made to order: new synthetic hormones give the win at any cost philosophy an even deadlier meaning in today's sports, by W. N. Taylor. PSYCHOLOGY TODAY 19(5):62-66, May 1985

Synthetic human growth hormone: a call for federal control, by W. N. Taylor. PHYSICIAN AND SPORTSMEDICINE 16(3):189-190+, March 1988

Use of human growth hormone poses a grave dilemma for sport, by T. Todd. SPORTS ILLUSTRATED 10-18, October 15, 1984
Todd summarizes remarks made by Dr. William J. Taylor at the National Convention of the American College of Sports medicine about somatotropin or human growth hormone. Taylor warns that parents are asking for growth hormone therapy to increase height in normal children even though results are questionable and possible side effects very dangerous. Both technical and slang terms are defined and explained.

Which children should have growth hormone therapy, by R. D. G. Milner. LANCET 8479:483-485, 1986
Not all short children respond to growth hormone therapy and existing criteria for diagnosis of growth hormone deficiency do not identify all children who can be made to grow faster with GH.

Side Effects

Anabolic androgenic steroids, synthetic derivatives of testosterone, can cause adverse side effects such as acne, balding, increased facial and body hair and voice deepening. Rare and more serious adverse effects, such as liver tumors, have been linked with the oral compounds when used in high doses for long periods. Aside from the physical risks, athletes experience psychological changes such as mood swings, violent behavior and rage while taking steroids and depression when they stop. This section includes references to both popular and professional articles on possible physical side effects to the liver, heart, arteries, etc., as well as the emotional problems associated with steroid use.

Side Effects: General

Adenocarcinoma of prostate in 40-year-old bodybuilder, by J. T. Roberts, et al. LANCET 2(8509):742, September 27, 1986

Adverse effects of anabolic steroids in athletes, by M. W. Kibble, et al. CLINICAL PHARMACY 6(9):686-692, September 1987

AIDS in a bodybuilder using anabolic steroids, by H. M. Sklarek, et al. NEW ENGLAND JOURNAL OF MEDICINE 311:1701, 1984

Anabolic androgenic steroids and a stroke in an athlete: case report, by M. A. Frankle, et al. ARCHIVES OF PHYSICAL MEDICINE AND REHABILITATION 69(8):632-633, August 1988
   This is a case report of a of 34-year-old bodybuilder with acute right hemiparesis and difficulty in speaking.

Anabolic steroids: to race against risk, by G. D. Braunstein. LOS ANGELES TIMES, October 9, 1988, Section V, p.3

Anabolics - part 3, by J. Wright. MUSCLE AND FITNESS 43(2):64-67+, February 1982

Androgenic steroid effects on serum hormones and on maximal force development in strength athletes, by M. Alen, et al. JOURNAL OF SPORTS MEDICINE AND PHYSICAL FITNESS 27(1):38-46, March 1987
   "The findings suggest that greater increases in muscular strength of the elite strength athletes occurred due to strength training with androgens rather than due to pure strength training."

Androgenic-anabolic steroid effects on serum thyroid, pituitary and steroid hormones in athletes, by M. Alen, et al. AMERICAN JOURNAL OF SPORTS MEDICINE 15(4):357-361, JULY/AUGUST 1987
    Endocrine responses in seven power athletes were studied during training period when the athletes were taking high doses of androgenic-anabolic steroids. Possible that abnormal findings in thyroid function tests may be found in athletes using steroids.

Are anabolic steroids for the long distance runner? ANNALS OF SPORTS MEDICINE 2(1):51-52, 1984

Athletes and steroids: playing a deadly game, by R. W. Miller. FDA CONSUMER 21(6):17-19+, November 1987
    This article briefly explains the physiology of testosterone in the body and lists prominent side effects. Topics also touched upon include women pumping iron, young users who don't want to be wimps, quack steroid products, NFL football players and cardiovascular/stroke problems.

Biological action of anabolic steroids: straight talk for coaches and educators. Les effets biologiques des steroides anabolisants, by L. J. Adams, et al. CAHPER JOURNAL/JOURNAL DE L'ACSEPL 55(2):32-36, March/April 1989

Concern rises on steroid use, a risky route for athletes, by H. M. Schmeck, Jr. NEW YORK TIMES, August 19, 1987, p. 42

Consequences of anabolic steroid abuse, by D. R. Lamb. SCHOLASTIC COACH 58(7):81, February 1989

Danger: athletes who are dying to win, steroids are potential killers; doctors who prescribe them should be prosecuted, by D. B. Riley. SCHOLASTIC COACH 54(4):48-50+, November 1984

Dead Russian athletes, by E. Mishara. OMNI 8(1):30, March 1986

Effect of anabolic treatment on the serum levels of gonadotropins, testosterone, prolactin, thyroid hormones and myoglobin of male athletes under physical training, by A. Clerico, et al. JOURNAL OF NUCLEAR MEDICINE AND ALLLIED SCIENCE 25(3):79-88, July/September 1981

Effects of anabolic steroids and strength training on the human immune response, by L. Calabrese, et al. MEDICINE AND SCIENCE IN SPORTS AND EXERCISE 21(4):386-392, August 1989
    The immune response was measured in steroid-using and non-steroid-using bodybuilders and the results indicated that (1) anabolic-androgenic steroid use as practiced by contemporary athletes is a powerful regulator of immune responsiveness and (2) autoantibodies are prevalent in strength-trained men even in the absence of anabolic steroid use. This is a technical article.

How sex hormones influence your fitness, Part 1, by L. Lamb. MUSCLE AND FITNESS 45(10):190-191, October 1984

Insulin resistance and diminished glucose tolerance in powerlifters ingesting anabolic steroids, by J. C. Cohen, et al. JOURNAL OF CLINICAL ENDOCRINOLOGY AND METABOLISM 64(5):960-963, May 1987

Jack King: drugs almost killed him, by B. Starr. IRON MAN 44(1):46-47+, November 1984

NSCA position paper on anabolic drug use by athletes. NSCA JOURNAL 7(4):27-31, 1985
This is a thorough discussion of the side effects of anabolic steroids.

Physical health and fitness of an elite bodybuilder during one year of administration of testosterone and anabolic steroids: a case study, by M. Alen, et al. INTERNATIONAL JOURNAL OF SPORTS MEDICINE 6(1):24-29, February 1985

Psychomotor and motor speed in power athletes self-administering testosterone and anabolic steroids, by P.Era, et al. RESEARCH QUARTERLY FOR EXERCISE AND SPORT 59:50-56, MARCH 1988

Response of serum hormones to androgen administration in power athletes, by M. Alen, et al. MEDICINE AND SCIENCE IN SPORTS AND EXERCISE 17(3):354-359, June 1985

Response of serum testosterone and its precursor steroids, SHBG and CBG, to anabolic steroid and testosterone self-administration in man, by A. Ruokonen et al. JOURNAL OF STEROID BIOCHEMISTRY 23(1):33-38, July 1985

Roids: the slow suicide, by B. Goldman. FLEX 2(9):56-57+, December 1984

Side effects from using steroids, by S. Burman, et al. MUSCLE AND FITNESS 50(10):28+, October 1989
Two doctors' observations on impotence in males and the relationship between steroids and psychiatric disorders are presented and specific case studies discussed.

Side effects of anabolic steroids in weight-trained men, by R. H. Strauss, et al. PHYSICIAN AND SPORTSMEDICINE 11(12):86-88+, December 1983

Spontaneous rupture of the extensor pollicis longus tendon after anabolic steroids, by M. Dramhoft, et al. JOURNAL OF HAND SURGERY 11(1):87, February 1986

Steroid abuse related to six athletes' deaths (including Daniel Baroudi). SPORTING NEWS 199:6, February 25, 1985

Strong medicine: in the controversy over anabolic steroids, little attention has been paid to their damaging, long-term effects, by A. Forsyth. SATURDAY NIGHT 99(5):15-17, May 1984

Study proposes to examine football players, powerlifters for possible long-term sequelae from anabolic steroid use in 1970's competition, by V. S. Cowart. JAMA 257(22):3021+, June 12, 1987
Study proposed to compare former steroid users with a matched 3025 control group of athletes who did not use them. Current health of the study population will be documented with attention to cardiovascular status, liver and endocrine function and psychological health.

Testicular responsiveness to human chorionic gonadotrophin during transient hypogonadotrophic hypogonadism induced by androgenic/anabolic steroids in power athletes, by H. Martikainen, et al. JOURNAL OF STEROID BIO-CHEMISTRY 25(1):109-112, July 1986

Testosterone: not for men only. Not simply a gender and growth factor, this vital hormone is linked to love, social behavior, criminality and even death, by F. C. Hatfield. MUSCLE AND FITNESS 44(9):36-37+, September 1983

Weighing the biological risks, by R. Price. MUSCLE AND FITNESS 45(2):91+, February 1984

Side Effects: Acne

Acne vulgaris in the athlete, by R. J. Conklin. PHYSICIAN AND SPORTSMEDI-CINE 16(10):57-60+, October 1988
    Anabolic-androgenic steroids are listed as one of many different aggre-vating factors for acne; (p.58-59), briefly mentions that some weight trainers and body builders may be tempted to use steroids and that they should be warned about acne as a possible side effect.

Effect of androgenic and anabolic steroids on the sebaceous gland in power athletes, by C. L. Kiraly, et al. ACTA DERMATO-VENEREOLOGICA 67(1): 36-40, 1987

Effect of testosterone and anabolic steroids on the size of sebaceous glands in power athletes, by C. L. Kiraly, et al. AMERICAN JOURNAL OF DERMATO-PATHOLOGY 9(6):515-509, December 1987

Side Effects: Gynecomastia

Consider the risks: mastectomy performed on man put on steroids by college athletic program, by C. Neff, et al. SPORTS ILLUSTRATED 66:7, January 26, 1987

Self-treatment of gynecomastia in bodybuilders who use anabolic steroids, by K. E. Friedl ,et al. PHYSICIAN AND SPORTSMEDICINE 17:67-71+, March 1989
    Some bodybuilders treat this feminizing side effect with additional drugs, i.e., androgens and HCG. Four case studies of bodybuilders are re-ported, one requiring mastectomy. Side effects such as breast pain and swelling only worsen with further steroid use. Author advises that ath-letes should be counseled to stop steroid use altogether. Self-administered drugs are not effective in reducing gynecomastia.

Surgical treatment of gynecomastia in the bodybuilder, by A. E. Aiache. PLASTIC AND RECONSTRUCTIVE SURGERY 83(1):61-66, January 1989

Side Effects: Heart

Acute myocardial infarction in a 22-year-old world class weight lifter using anabolic steroids, by R. A. McNutt , et al. AMERICAN JOURNAL OF CARDIOLOGY 62(1):164, July 1, 1988

Are anabolics atherogenic?, by W. N. Taylor. STRENGTH AND HEALTH 52(6): 69-61, October/November 1984
> This article summarizes more than just the "artery clogging" effects, including psychological facets, i.e., mental intensity which may turn inward to overstress the heart.

Increased left ventricular mass in a bodybuilder using anabolic steroids, by G. McKillop, et al. BRITISH JOURNAL OF SPORTS MEDICINE 29(4):151-152, December 1986

Left ventricular size and function in bodybuilders using anabolic steroids, by R. C. Salke, et al. MEDICINE AND SCIENCE IN SPORTS AND EXERCISE 17(6): 701-704, December 1985

Levels of serum sex hormones and risk factors for coronary heart disease in exercise-trained men, by B. Gutin, et al. AMERICAN JOURNAL OF MEDICINE 79(1):79-84, July 1985

Was the X factor a factor?, by S. Courson. SPORTS ILLUSTRATED 70:34, April 3, 1989

Side Effects: Lipoproteins/Cholesterol

Alphalipoproteinemic effects of androgenic-anabolic steroids in athletes, by D. M. Crist, et al. ANNALS OF SPORTS MEDICINE 2(3):125-128, 1985

Anabolic-androgenic steroid effects on endocrinology and lipid metabolism in athletes, by M. Alen, et al. SPORTS MEDICINE 6(6):327-332, 1988
> This article reviews current research studies on the biological actions of synthetic anabolic-androgenic steroids on endocrinology and lipid metabolism and their interactions during training.

Androgenic-anabolic steroid effects on serum and skin surface lipids, on red cells and on liver enzymes, by C. L. Kiraly. INTERNATIONAL JOURNAL OF SPORTS MEDICINE 9(4):249-252, August 1988
> The effects of large doses of testosterone and anabolic steroids on the serum lipids and skin surface lipids were studied during a 12-week strength training period. Decreased serum high-density lipoprotein cholesterol (HDLC) and elevated serum triglyceride levels were found at the same time with an elevated skin surface lipid cholesterol level.

Androgens reduce HDL2-cholesterol and increase hepatic triglyceride lipase activity, by M. A. Kantor, et al. MEDICINE AND SCIENCE IN SPORTS AND EXERCISE 17(4):462-465, August 1985

Deleterious effects of anabolic steroid on serum lipoproteins, blood pressure and liver function in amateur bodybuilders, by J. W. Lenders . INTERNATIONAL JOURNAL OF SPORTS MEDICINE 9(1):19-23, February 1988
> The effects of self-administered anabolic steroids (AS) on lipoproteins, liver function and blood pressure were studied in male amateur bodybuilders. Twenty bodybuilders were studied at the end of a course of AS(group 1) and 42 bodybuilders were studied after discontinuation of the AS for a mean of 5 months (group 2). Sixteen bodybuilders were studied after discontinuation of AS for at least 2 months and at the end of a 9-week course of AS (group 3). A groups of 13 bodybuilders who never used AS served as a control group.

Exercise training, sex hormones, and lipoprotein relationships in men, by M. A. Frey, et al. JOURNAL OF APPLIED PHYSIOLOGY: RESPIRATORY, ENVIRONMENTAL AND EXERCISE PHYSIOLOGY 54(3):757-762, March 1983

> This study sought to determine whether changes in high density lipoprotein cholesterol (HDLC) could be mediated by changes in endogenous testosterone and estrogen occurring during exercise training in men. The results suggest changes in endogenous testosterone and estrogens may mediate the increases in HDLC reported after exercise training programs in men.

High-density-lipoprotein cholesterol in bodybuilders v. powerlifters: negative effects of androgen use, by B. F. Hurley, et al. JAMA 252(4):507-513, July 27, 1984

> Eight bodybuilders and four powerlifters were tested before and after androgen use to evaluate the effects of anabolic-androgenic steroids on lipids and the relationship to type of weight training. Androgen use by the bodybuilders and power lifters lowered values of both HDL-Cholesterol and HDL2-C by 55 percent and raised values of LDL-C 6 percent and LDL-CHDL-C ratios 280 percent. The training regimen of bodybuilders is associated with a more favorable lipid profile than the training use by powerlifters.

Hypercholesterolemia in male power lifters using anabolic-androgenic steroids, by J. C. Cohen, et al. PHYSICIAN AND SPORTSMEDICINE 16(8), 49-50+, August 1988

> Serum total cholesterol (TC) concentrations were measured in three groups of male power lifters who used anabolic-androgenic steroids; 19 who used steroids for eight weeks, seven of the 19 who continued steroid use for three years, and three who had been using steroids for eight years.

Lipoprotein analysis in bodybuilders, by G. McKillop, et al. INTERNATIONAL JOURNAL OF CARDIOLOGY 17(3):281-288, December 1987

Marked fall in high-density lipoprotein following isotretinoin therapy, by G. N. Hoag, et al. JOURNAL OF THE AMERICAN ACADEMY OF DERMATOLOGY 16(6):1264-1265, June 1987

> This article reports the case of a weightlifter on anabolic steroids.

Physiological performance, serum hormones, enzymes and lipids of an elite power athlete during training with and without androgens during prolonged detraining, by K. Haekkinen, et al. JOURNAL OF SPORTS MEDICINE AND PHYSICAL FITNESS 26(1):92-100, March 1986

Reduced high-density lipoprotein-cholesterol in power athletes: use of male sex hormone derivatives, an atherogenic factor, by M. Alen, et al. INTERNATIONAL JOURNAL OF SPORTS MEDICINE 5(6):341-342, December 1984

> The effect of androgenic steroids on plasma lipids was studied in seven power athletes who self-administered androgenic steroids on the average of 45 mg/day during an 8-week strength training period. At the beginning of the study, no significant differences were noticed in HDL-cholesterol by 54% (1.47 to 0.67 mmol/1).

Serum lipids in power athletes self-administering testosterone and anabolic steroids, by M. Alen, et al. INTERNATIONAL JOURNAL OF SPORTS MEDICINE 6(3):139-144, June 1985

Study: steroids lower immunity, lipids. PHYSICIAN AND SPORTSMEDICINE 16(2):56+, February 1988

Side Effects: Liver

Androgenic steroid effects on liver and red cells, by M. Alen. BRITISH JOURNAL OF SPORTS MEDICINE 19(1):15-20, March 1985

Hepatic neoplasms associated with contraceptive and anabolic steroids, by K. G. Ishak. RECENT STUDIES IN CANCER RESEARCH 66:73-128, 1979
    This lengthy article reviews reports of malignant tumors of the liver in patients using oral contraceptives or anabolic steroids after first explaining and showing the differences between focal modular hyperplasia and hepatocellular adenoma, benign tumors of the liver, using extensive photomicrographs.

Hepatic tumours induced by anabolic steroids in an athlete, by T. M. Creagh, et al. JOURNAL OF CLINICAL PATHOLOGY 41(4):441-443, April 1988

Severe liver diseases possibly associated with anabolic steroids, by W. Taylor. MUSCLE DIGEST 8(4):8+, August 1984

Side Effects: Psychological

Affective and psychotic symptoms associated with anabolic steroid use, by H. G. Pope, et al. AMERICAN JOURNAL OF PSYCHIATRY 145(4):487-490, April 1988
    Structured interviews were performed with 41 bodybuilders and football players who used anabolic steroids in order to assess the frequency of affective and psychotic symptoms.

Anabolic steroids and acute schizophrenic episode, by W. J. Annitto, et al. JOURNAL OF CLINICAL PSYCHIATRY 41(4):143-144
    This is a case report of a male high school senior who developed an acute schizophreni form illness in 1978 after using anabolic steroids in 1977 and 1978 while weight lifting to "gain weight." Authors alert physicians that there is a possibility of a schizophrenic-like reaction in an athlete ingesting anabolic steroids.

Anabolic-androgenic steroid dependence, by K. J. Brower, et al. JOURNAL OF CLINICAL PSYCHIATRY 50(1):31-33, January 1989
    Presents the case of a 24-year-old man whose dependence on a combination of steroids caused mood disturbance and marital conflict.

Bodybuilder's psychosis: anabolic steroids. NURSE'S DRUG ALERT 11(7):54-55, July 1987
    Two men were hospitalized with first-time psychotic eppisodes associated with symptoms of severe depression. One, a 40-year-old, had been taking the androgen methyltestosterone, 10 mg bid, for two weeks as a treatment for idiopathic impotence. The other, aged 22, was a bodybuilder who had recently completed his second eight-week course of methandrostenolone, 15 mg/day. In both men, medical and neuroendocrine findings were unremarkable.

Does steroid abuse cause or excuse violence? by A. Lubell. PHYSICIAN AND SPORTS MEDICI NE 17:176-185, February 1989
Lubell examines steroid dependence as a legal defense for violent crime.

Final word on steroids, by D. Geringer. RUNNER'S WORLD 19(8):144-146+, August 1984

Insanity of steroid abuse: the drug can give athletes major mental problems, by T. Monmaney. NEWSWEEK 111:75, May 23, 1988

Male madness: steroids and the risk of testosterone poisoning, by J. Jerome. OUTSIDE 10(8):25-26+, August 1985

Mean mental muscles: the psychological price of steroids, by J. Slothower. HEALTH 20:1, January 1988

Nightmare of steroids, by T. Chaikin, et al. SPORTS ILLUSTRATED 69(18):82-88+, October 24, 2988
South Carolina lineman Tommy Chaikin used bodybuilding drugs for three years. They drove him to violence and nearly to suicide.

Of muscles and mania, by E. Grant. PSYCHOLOGY TODAY 21:12, September 1987

Psychological problem patterns found with athletes, by S. R. Heyman. CLINICAL PSYCHOLOGIST 39(3):68-71, Summer 1986
This article describes common problems found in working with athletes including alcohol and drug abuse and physical aggression and suggests developing controls that allow expression of aggression in the athletic arena but not in other domains of life.

Psychosis cited from steroid use, by V. Cohn. WASHINGTON POST, August 4, 1987, p. 5

Steroids' side effects: depression, paranoia. SPORT 79:17, February 1988

Steroids stir mental backlash: psychiatric complications caused by athletes' use of steroids. SCIENCE NEWS 133:284, April 30, 1988

Testing and Drug Enforcement

This section lists popular and professional articles on drug testing, black market availability of anabolic steroids and growth hormone, FDA crackdown on suppliers and pushers and other related drug control problems and legal issues.

Testing: General

Abuse of hormone drugs in sport, by R.V. Brooks. ANALYTICAL PROCEED-INGS 24(3):70-71, 1987
> Brief overview with specific testing methods explained . . . sensitive indicators of testosterone doping.

Accord on drug testing, sanctions sought before 1992 Olympics in Europe. JAMA 260:3397-3398, December 16, 1988
> International Olympic Committee approved an international charter aimed at controlling drug abuse . . . drug testing must be done at random.

Anabolic actions, by R. Sullivan, et al. SPORTS ILLUSTRATED 64:13, April 21, 1986

Analytical chemistry at the Games of the XXIIIrd Olympiad in Los Angeles, 1984, by D. H. Catlin, et al. CLINICAL CHEMISTRY 33(2):319-327, February 1987

Athlete disputes the fairness of mandatory testing for drugs, by K. Schmidt. SPORTS ILLUSTRATED 64(16):9, April 21, 1986

Banning drugs in sports: a skeptical view, by N. Fost. HASTINGS CENTER REPORT 16(4):5-10, August 1986
> Author says/feels that there is not a clear distinction between therapeutic drugs used for injury or pain control and the illegal drugs like anabolic steroids.

Bosworth faces the music: Brian Bosworth was a conspicuous casualty of the NCAA's steroid crackdown, by C. Neff. SPORTS ILLUSTRATED 66(1):20-22+, January 5, 1987

Bridging the gap—research: anabolic steroid detection, by M. G. Di-Pasquale. NATIONAL STRENGTH AND CONDITIONING ASSOCIATION JOURNAL 10(2):26-27, April/May 1988

British expands drug-testing program beyond competition: includes testing during training. NEW YORK TIMES 1:14, November 11, 1987

Chemical corner: steroid testing update, by J. Everson. MUSCLE AND FITNESS 47(6):135-137, June 27, 1986

Colleges learn that testing athletes for steroids won't be easy or cheap. CHRONI-CLE OF HIGHER EDUCATION 30:27-28, May 8, 1985

Colleges must clean up their athletics programs or face professionalization, NCAA President says, by C. S. Farrell. CHRONICLE OF HIGHER EDUCATION 33 (37):27-28, May 27, 1987
 Wilford S. Bailey of Auburn University is heading the National Collegiate Athletic Association as it strugggles to cope with several controversial issues: testing athletes for drug abuse, new academic standards for freshman athletes, the role of college presidents in governing sports and the integrity of college athletics.

Congress considers ban on mail-order steroids. PHYSICIAN AND SPORTS-MEDICINE 17(5):34+, May 1989

Congressman looks at steroids, by R. H. Baker. ATHLETIC ADMINISTRATION 22:13+, November 1987

Detection and quantitation of methandienone: Dianabol, in urine by isotope dilution—mass fragmentography, by I. Bjorkhem, et al. JOURNAL OF STEROID BIOCHEMISTRY 13(2):169-175, February 1980
 This is a very technical discussion of results of sample testing of urine with a highly accurate method developed for detection and quantitation of methadienone: Dianabol, one of the most widely used anabolic steroids.

Detection of anabolic steroid administration to athletes, by R. V. Brooks, et al. JOURNAL OF STEROID BIOCHEMISTRY 11(1):913-917, July 1979
 This is a technical article about the detection of the main synthetic anabolic steroids by radioimmunoassay screening. The authors also investigate the possibility of detecting the administration of the natural androgen testosterone.

Detection of androgenic anabolic steroids in urine, by C. K. Hatton, et al. CLINI-CAL LABORATORY MEDICINE 7(3):655-668, September 1987

Drug cheaters may be winning battle with testers, by M. Janofsky. NEW YORK TIMES, September 15, 1988, p.53
 Olympic athletes are said to mask steroid use, subverting drug tests.

Drug of champions, by E. Marshall. SCIENCE 242(4876):183-184, October 14, 1988
 Good review and discussion is provided on the black market and testing.

Drug testing. LEGAL MEMORANDUM:9, October 1987
 A number of legal issues are involved in conducting a drug testing pro-gram to determine whether students—and occasionally teachers—are using illegal drugs. Two legal issues have been raised concerning the ac-curacy of the urinalysis test: whether it is chemically accurate and whether appropriate procedures have been followed to make certain that the tests apply to the right specimen.

Drug testing and the games, by R. E. Leach. SKIING 36(6):30-31+, February 1984

Drug testing in a university athletic program: protocol and implementation, by G. D. Rovere, et al. PHYSICIAN AND SPORTSMEDICINE 14(4):69-74+, April 1986
>An athletic drug education, counseling and screening program at Wake Forest University is described. Decisions regarding which athletes to test, which drugs to test for and how to test for them, how to collect urine samples and measures taken for a positive result are discussed.

Drug testing of athletes: test the team's pooled urine, by F. R. Dixon, et al. JAMA 262(9), September 1, 1989
>The letter writer suggests pooling urine from every one on the team and if the pooled urine is tainted, the team would lose its event. Such an approach would build peer pressure against drug use while protecting individual privacy says the writer.

Drug testing programs face snags and legal challenges, by V. S. Cowart. PHYSICIAN-AND-SPORTSMEDICINE 16(2):165-167, February 1988

Drugged and victorious: doping in sport, by P. Sperryn. NEW SCIENTIST 1415: 16-19, August 2, 1984
>We spend large sums of money testing athletes for drugs, yet doping is still commonplace. An international revolt against the present system of drug control is gathering momentum.

Drugs: a moment of pleasure for a lifetime of pain, by S. Feldman. COACHING VOLLEYBALL 1(6):31, August/September 1988

Fralic frets over steroids. SPORTING NEWS 202:37, October 27, 1986

Getting serious about steroids, by R. Heitzinger. ATHLETIC BUSINESS11:32-35, September 1987
>This article reflects the different opinions about the seriousness of drug testing for steroids as opposed to recreational drugs such as cocaine. The NCAA drug testing progress is introduced, costs of random testing dis-cussed, and the reasons some athletes continue to use steroids despite health risks explained.

Hormones under medical control?, by K. Hartiala. OLYMPIC REVIEW 175:263-264, May 1982
>This is a brief opinion paper that argues in favor of improved doping control also during the training period and against allowing the use of certain hormones even under medical supervision.

International drug charter gains approval, by M. Janofsky. NEW YORK TIMES, November 25, 1988, p. B10

In the news: random drug testing. CURRENT HEALTH 2(14):26, May 1988

Marathoner returns to save name, by M. Moran. NEW YORK TIMES November 3, 1988, p.A47
>Antoni Niemczak to run in New York City Marathon.

NCAA approves drug testing of players at football bowl games, championships, by P. Monaghan. CHRONICLE OF HIGHER EDUCATION 31(19):29+, January 22, 1986

NCAA does off-season testing for steroids, by M. Duda. PHYSICIAN AND SPORTSMEDICINE 16(4):49, April 1988

Olympic drug bust, by R. Virtanen, et al. RUNNERS WORLD 19(12):80-83+, December 1984
> A test for banned substances cost Finnish star Martti Vainio his medal in the 10,000 and cast his homeland into mourning. He admitted to B-12 injections, but not to the knowledge that they contained steroids.

Olympics drug testing: basis for future study, by P. Gunby. JAMA 252(4):454-455+, July 27, 1984
> This article provides an excellent overview of the topic highlighting consideration of the drug control question by the U/S Olympic Committee's (USOC) Sports Medicine Division, as well as athletes' rights in the matter of testing . . . advised when drug testing could lead to punitive action . . . how athletes are attempting cheating.

Positive step, by S. Wulf. SPORTS ILLUSTRATED 69:25, November 7, 1988
> NFL to treat steroid use the same as cocaine abuse.

Practical aspects of screening of anabolic steroids in doping control with particular accent to nortestosterone radioimmunoassay using mixed antisera, by R. Hampl, et al. JOURNAL OF STEROID BIOCHEMISTRY 11(10):933-936, July 1979

Problems of oral contraceptives in dope control of anabolic steroids, by D. DeBoer, et al. BIOMEDICAL AND ENVIRONMENTAL MASS SPECTROMETRY 17(2):127-128, August 1988

Reversing field, by C. Neff. SPORTS ILLUSTRATED 64:15, December 8, 1986
> NFL to test for anabolic steroids.

Squeezing the drugs from athletics. INSIGHT 46-47, December 26, 1988-January 2, 1989
> This is a discussion of random testing from an international perspective. Scandinavian countries already conduct such tests, West Germany soon will and Bulgaria is planning random testing. U. S. and Soviet Union are considering off-season testing of each other's athletes.

Steroid hormones in sports. Special reference: sex hormones and their derivatives, by M. T. Lucking. INTERNATIONAL JOURNAL OF SPORTS MEDICINE 3(Suppl)1:65-67, February 1982

Steroid justice, by C. Neff. SPORTS ILLUSTRATED 63(11):11, December 9, 1985

Steroid Task Force completes report. NATIONAL FEDERATION NEWS 7(2):14, October 1989

Steroids and the law: what does your state penal code say about anabolic steroids?, by L. Uzych. MUSCLE FITNESS 50(2):118-119+, February 1989

Steroids: another view, by S. Courson. SPORTS ILLUSTRATED 69(21):106, November 14, 1988
> All we can do, this former player argues, is monitor usage.

Stoned on ice. ECONOMIST 306:91-92, February 13, 1988

Stopping anabolic steroid abuse on a zero dollar budget, by D. Wathen. NATION-
AL STRENGTH AND CONDITIONING ASSOCIATION JOURNAL 10:56-60,
December1988/January 1989
   Run tests on individuals suspected and offer rehabilitation. Sign a waiver
   to submit to unannounced drug screens through urinalysis.

Strength and weakness, by S. Wulf. SPORTS ILLUSTRATED 66:21, June 1,
1987
   Steroid ring busted; NCAA testing program called ineffective.

Strides against steroids: The athletics congress plans year-round random drug
testing, by S. Wulf. SPORTS ILLUSTRATED 70:19, June 26, 1989

Summaries of changes in regulations approves by the NCAA convention.
CHRONICLE OF HIGHER EDUCATION 31(19):34-35, January 22, 1986

System accused of failing test posed by drugs, by M. Janofsky, et al. NEW YORK
TIMES. November 17, 1988, p. A1

Testy: Athletics congress announces drug testing at pepsi invitational, shot put
and discus cancelled due to withdrawals, by S. Wulf. SPORTS ILLUS-
TRATED 64:14, May 30, 1988

Text of American Council's draft guidelines on testing athletes for drugs. CHRO-
NICLE OF HIGHER EDUCATION 32(10):34, May 7, 1986
   The text of the American Council on Education's draft proposed guidelines for drug testing of college athletes is provided with the suggestion
   that such programs should be used to prevent use of performance-
   enhancing drugs that undermine the integrity of athletic competition.

Tricks of the trade, by C. Neff. SPORTS ILLUSTRATED 70:8, February 13, 1989
   Canadian weighlifters suspended from Olympics took painful measures
   to mask their steroid use.

Two bills on steroid use. NEW YORK TIMES 1:10, March 1, 1989

US, USSR join forces to combat steroid use, by M. Duda. PHYSICIAN AND
SPORTSMEDICINE 17(8):16+, August 1989
   This "newsbrief," introducing the US-Soviet antidoping pact . . . "intended to demonstrate that two countries can work together successfully to
   control doping," reports that both sides gave good cooperation and
   financial backing.

Uses, abuses and detection of anabolic steroids, by P. Gains. ATHLETICS 8-11,
May 1982
   After a review of steroid hormones, brief discussion of medical uses, use
   by athletes, and adverse reactions to steroids. The author explains the
   development of testing procedures; identifies steroid takers who had
   been caught from 1975-1981 and reports in some detail the case of
   Alexis Paul- MacDonald, a Canadian athlete who tested positive, but
   denied taking anabolic steroids.

Varying standards on steroid use, by W. C. Rhoden. NEW YORK TIMES October
2, 1988, p.E9
   Disparity between amateur and professional sports groups is discussed.

Who tests which athletes for what drugs?, by M. Duda. PHYSICIAN AND
    SPORTS MEDICINE 16:155-161, February 1988
        This article reviews trends in drug testing policies and procedures, includ-
        ing which drugs are tested, when tests are conducted, and penalties for
        those who test positive.

Why ban drugs?, by S. Baddeley. BADMINTON NOW 4(56):16-18, February
    1988

Will drug testing in sports play for industry?, by J. W. Hoffman, et al. PERSONNEL
    JOURNAL 66(5):52-59, May 1987
        This article seems to be more directed at cocaine and heroin misuse, but
        issues on drug testing are appropriate to anabolic steroids too.

Will the polygraph eliminate steroids?, by R. O'Brien. MUSCLE AND FITNESS
    49:29+, November 1988

Testing: the Black Market

California proposes tougher steroid law, by M. Duda. PHYSICIAN AND SPORTS-
    MEDICINE 14(2):40, February 1986

Charges in steroid case. NEW YORK TIMES. December 9, 1988, p.B16

Confessions of a steroid smuggler, by J. Eisendrath. MUSCLE AND FITNESS 49:
    158-160+, 1988
        This is William Dillon's story of being one of the biggest dealers of black
        market anabolic steroids based in the San Diego area and smuggling
        drugs from Mexico, he cooperated with federal authorities and was await-
        ing sentencing at the time the article was written.

For athletes and dealers, black market steroids are risky business. FDA CON-
    SUMER 21(7):24-25, SEPTEMBER 1987

Muscling in, by S. Penn. WALL STREET JOURNAL 212:1+, October 4, 1988.
        As ever more people try anabolic steroids, traffickers take over; dope
        dealers smuggle drugs from Mexico for athletes and for the merely vain;
        sideline business at the gym.

On the black market, drugs are in easy reach of public, by P. Alfano, et al. NEW
    YORK TIMES . November 18, 1988, p. A1
        This article includes a related article on description of steroids.

People helper, by C. Neff, et al. SPORTS ILLUSTRATED 63:26, December 23,
    1985
        Richard "Tony" Fitton sentenced for trafficking steroids to college ath-
        letes.

Some predict increased steroid use in sports despite drug testing, crackdown on
    suppliers, by V. Cowart. JAMA 257(22):3025+,June 12, 1987
        Yesalis and Wright, both authors and researchers on steroid use, are re-
        ported as expecting steroid use to increase despite NCAA testing be-
        cause powerlifters, bodybuilders and football players all see the benefits
        outweighing the risks. A brief reporting of testing challenges introduces
        the privacy issue.

Steroid ring broken; ex-Olympian held (David Jenkins), by J. Schachter. LOS
ANGELES TIMES. May 22, 1987, Section I,p.3

Steroid underground, by D. Nassif. MUSCLE AND FITNESS 45(2):92-93,
February 1984

Testing: Classification as Controlled Substances

Classifying steroid as controlled substances suggested to decrease athletes'
supply, but enforcement could be a major problem, by V. Cowart. JAMA
257(22):3029, June 12, 1987
This reports that William Taylor, physician and author, recommends that
steroids be classified as controlled substances and warns of personality
changes that some steroid users develop. Taylor also warns that steroid
use by young persons will have powerful effects on maturation and
stature.

Controlling the supply of anabolic steroids, by R. H. Strauss. PHYSICIAN AND
SPORTS MEDICINE 15(5): 41, May 1987

Synthetic anabolic-androgenic steroids: a plea for controlled substance status, by
W. N. Taylor. PHYSICIAN AND SPORTSMEDICINE 15(5):140-148+, May
1987

Would controlled substance status affect steroid trafficking?, by V. S. Cowart.
PHYSICIAN AND SPORTSMEDICINE 15(5):151-152+, May 1987

Testing: Legal Issues

Analysis of public college athlete drug testing programs through the unconsti-
tutional condition doctrine and the fourth amendment, by S. L. Meloch.
SOUTHERN CALIFORNIA LAW REVIEW 60:815-850, March 1987
After an introduction to the problem of drugs and sports, the author
examines the fourth amendment in relation to student-athletes and
considers whether drug tests are an illegal search and seizure. Author
argues that the individual's right to privacy outweigh the school's need for
drug testing. Extensive legal references are cited and an actual sample
consent form duplicated

Constitutionality of mandatory student-athlete drug testing programs: the bounds
of privacy, by E. Lock, et al. UNIVERSITY OF FLORIDA LAW REVIEW 38:
581-613, Fall 1986
This article reviews the legal challenges that NCAA and college/university
drug testing programs face: right to privacy, random drug testing in the
absence of suspicion, etc. It is recommended that programs stress education and treatment. Steroids are specifically mentioned on pages 601-
602 in a discussion of drug screens, particular drugs, and performance.
Extensive legal and other references on drug testing are provided and
discussed.

Does the National Collegiate Athletic Associations' Drug Testing Program test
positive if it is subjected to constitutional scrutiny?, by J. V. Fonti. DRAKE
LAW REVIEW 37:83-102, 1987-1988

After a brief introduction to some statistics on drug usage in general, this article discusses the N.C.A.A.'s drug testing program and the possible legal challenges based on the fourth amendment, bill of rights. Urinalysis is compared to the taking of blood as a highly invasive search. Random drug testing as opposed to testing based upon reasonable suspicion is argued against.

Drug testing: the toughest competition an athlete ever faces, by E. Dobberstein. THURGOOD MARSHALL LAW REVIEW 13:143-160, Fall/Spring 1987-1988
This article reviews the history of drug testing among amateur athletes and then discusses the constitutional issues that drug testing involves ranging from the right to privacy to equal protection. Student-athletes cannot look to a uniform standard throughout the country and they are afforded less protection, the author concludes, than other citizens.

Drug testing in professional and college sports, by L. M. Rose. UNIVERSITY OF KANSAS LAW REVIEW 36:787-821, Summer 1988
This article provides a very thorough and well documented review of drug use by athletes; discusses why athletes use drugs; reviews the testing procedures and practices in the National Football League, National Basketball Association, Major League Baseball, other professional sports and college athletics; and discusses lawsuits and other problems raised by drug testing of college athletes. Steroids are specifically mentioned in the discussions of drug use, NCAA testing and challenges to amateur drug testing (pp. 789, 791, 812, 813, 818, 820).

Drug testing in sports, by S. F. Brock, et al. DICKINSON LAW REVIEW 92:505-570, Spring 1988
This is a very thorough and technical overview of the arguments for and against drug testing of athletes, an examination of programs and discussion of legal challenges. Specific professional sports (horse racing, boxing, baseball, football, basketball and hockey) are covered as well as amateur sports, the NCAA, and the University of Washington's drug testing program. Privacy claims, confidentiality, contractual disputes, and specific cases are cited and discussed. Authors conclude that for amateur athletes drug testing should be permitted only where voluntary, based on reasonable cause, and the sport is dangerous.

Drug testing of athletes and the United States Constitution: Crisis and conflict, by J. O. Cochran. DICKINSON LAW REVIEW 92:571-607, Spring 1988

Drug, athletes and the NCAA: A proposed rule for mandatory drug testing in college athletics, by J. B. Ford. JOHN MARSHALL LAW REVIEW 18:205-236 Fall 1984
The author discusses the need for a drug-testing rule in college athletics and comments on the constitutional problems such as privacy considerations that might be used to challenge the NCAA action. Extensive legal and other references concerning drug used by athletes are offered. Steroids are specifically mentioned (p 231) as one of the specific performance-enhancing drugs which can harm athletes and thus should be tested for use.

Mandatory drug testing in sports: the law in Canada, by J. Trossman. UNIVERSITY OF TORONTO FACULTY OF LAW REVIEW 47:191-219, Fall 1988
After a review of drug-related incidents and deaths of famous Canadian and American athletes, the author comments on the legal constraints on drug testing of professional athletes in Canada. Steroids are mentioned

in the first few pages related to the Ben Johnson scandal, but the discussion focuses on drugs that clearly hamper performance rather than drugs that appear to enhance performance. Extensive discussion of legal challenges to mandatory drug testing is offered and arguments provided.

Mandatory drug testing of college athletes: are athletes being denied their constitutional rights?, by A. Rose. PEPPERDINE LAW REVIEW 16:45-75, December 1988

> After a brief review of drug abuse and doping in sports, the author comments on mandatory drug testing programs implemented by the NCAA and individual universities and colleges in light of the fourth amendment protection against unreasonable searches and seizures and the athlete's right to privacy. Includes an appendix of NCAA banned drug classes, 1987-1988. Many legal references are cited under the fourth amendment challenge.

NCAA declares war: student-athletes battle the mandatory drug test, by R. J. Meredith. CAPITAL UNIVERSITY LAW REVIEW 16:673-700, Summer 1987

> After reviewing the benefits and defects of mandatory drug testing program, the author analyses the legality of mandatory urinalysis testing based on case law and challenges to employer mandatory drug testing. Then the author discusses the NCAA drug testing program and that which was developed at Ohio State University. Anabolic steroids are specifically discussed on pages 675-676 under the benefit of mandatory drug testing because it would deter athletes from using steroids, thereby promoting the athlete's safety by avoiding inherent risks and because testing will ensure fairness to all athletes by putting users and non-users on equal grounds in terms of strength and weight.

Playing the drug-testing game: college athletes, regulatory institutions, and the structures of constitutional argument, by J. A. Scanlan. INDIANA LAW JOURNAL 62:863-983, 1986-1987

Random urinalysis: Violating the athlete's individual rights?, by D. L. Ayers. HOWARD LAW JOURNAL 30:93-142, 1987

> After a fine introduction to drug abuse in general, the author comments that athletes are expected to conform to higher standards of personal conduct then the general public and yet the pressure to excel tempts athletes to use drugs to enhance performance and gain a competitive edge. The author goes on to discuss the drug testing agreements in professional sports: tennis, basketball, football, and baseball. Then a constitutional analysis and arguments against random testing for professional athletes is provided, including ethical considerations.

Training Alternatives

This section lists articles on dietary supplements and strength training regimens that do not involve anabolic steroids: anti-catabolic training (A.C.T.), resistance, amino acids, hypnosis and mental imagery.

A.C.T.: the steroid alternative, by T. V. Pipes. SCHOLASTIC COACH 57(6):106+, January 1988
>The author, a former steroid user, presents a training program that reduces the destructive forces in training, catabolic metabolism; he provides ten guidelines to be followed. He then explains why his strength training program works to build up muscle protein and thus gain physicial size and strength.

Amino acid supplements: beneficial or risky?, by J. L. Slavin, et al. PHYSICIAN AND SPORTS MEDICINE 16(3):221-222+, March 1988
>It has never been proven that amino acid supplements can benefit endurance athletes or bodybuilders who are in good health and are consuming adequate diets. There is some discussion of growth hormones. Arginine and ornithine have a significant effect but some potential risks and costs outrageously overpriced. Amino acid supplements are just expensive and unneeded protein supplements.

Amino acids—the effective muscle builder, by P. Mardle. THROWER 35: 21-22, May 1986

Analysis of the relationship between "psychical impetus" and physiology among competitive athletes, by A. J. Hoffman. INTERNATIONAL JOURNAL OF SPORT PSYCHOLOGY 14(4):270-281, 1983
>The presence of "psychical impetus," which is defined by the author as an increased or added psychological strength that actually influences physical strength otherwise thought to be absent in the individual, was tested. The overall experimental design was a 2-trial sequence followed by a postexperimental interview. It is concluded that as psychical impetus develops, an increase in heart rate and amount of weight used in the benchpress task significantly increases.

Changes in the self concept and athletic performance of weight lifters through a cognitive-hypnotic approach: an empirical study, by W. Howard, et al. AMERICAN JOURNAL OF CLINICAL HYPNOSIS 28(4):248-257, April 1986
>This study examined the effects of a cognitive-hypnotic-imagery approach (CHI), cognitive restructuring, and hypnosis only treatments on neuromuscular performance, muscular growth, reduction of anxiety and enhancement of self-concept in 32 male weightlifters (mean age 22.5 yrs). Data suggest that combining hypnotic relaxation and imagery with

cognitive restructuring enhances both the immediate and long-range effects of treatment.

Combating chemical warfare: ergogenic aids in sports, by C. E. Percy. SPORTS-MEDICINE DIGEST 4(11):4-5, November 1982

Effects of a commercial dietary supplement on human performance, by D. W. Barnett, et al. AMERICAN JOURNAL OF CLINICAL NUTRITION 40(3):586-590, September 1984

> Twenty male runners were tested as to whether a commercial ergogenic supplement was of any physiological benefit to their endurance performance. Either a placebo or the supplement (a vitamin, mineral, amino acid and unsaturated fatty acid complex) was administered to the subjects daily over a 4-week period in a double-blind design. The authors conclude that the supplement had no beneficial effect on performance as indicated by its inability to alter significantly any of the metabolic or physiological parameters, and that supplements of this nature are of no physiological value to the athlete who consumes a normal nutritionally balanced diet.

Effects of hydraulic-resistance strength training on serum lipid levels in prepubertal boys, by A. Weltman, et al. AMERICAN JOURNAL OF DISEASES OF CHILDREN 141(7): 777-780, July 1987

Energizing way to weight train: split routines, by M. Greenwood-Robinson. WOMEN'S SPORTS AND FITNESS 41-43, July/August 1989

> This article proposes training only one, two or three major muscle groups-legs, chest, back, etc. - at a time in each work out. Sample schedules are provided for three-to-six day routines.

Ergogenic aids, by E. F. Coyle. CLINICS IN SPORTS MEDICINE 3(3):731-742, July 1984

> The effectiveness of various ergogenic aids for improving physical performance is discussed. Specific topics include carbohydrate supplementation during exercise and fat utilization, as well as methods of reducing the accumulation of metabolic by-products (that is, heat and acid) and increasing muscular strength.

Essentials of nutrition for athletes, by M. N. Volgarey, et al. SOVIET SPORTS REVIEW 22(3):114-118, September 1987

> This article provides an overview of effective nutrition of a healthy man and its essentials in sport participation. It includes a table of daily energy requirements of athletes (protein, fat, carbohydrates, calories) by sport. It also reports that athletes' need for protein increases in the period of training, but not for extreme increases. There is a negative effect of overloading on the liver and kidney.

Facts of resistance training, by M. Kemp. MODERN ATHLETE AND COACH 27(2):37-40, April 1989

> The author introduces the three most common forces that an athlete in track and field has to overcome: gravity, friction and the drag of air resistance. Kemp explains that resistance training develops strength, power and endurance and suggests specific strength development exercises. He also defines performance terminology such as: maximum strength, speed strength, strength endurance and hypertrophy.

Getting bigger, but by-passing steroids: amino acid alternative, by K. Szkalak. MUSCLE DIGEST 4(5):60-61+, October 1980

How much protein does an athlete need?, by D. K. Layman. PHYSICIAN AND SPORTS MEDICINE 15(12):181-183, December 1987
This article explains the physiology of protein digestion in the human body. Protein needs for muscle growth are small—excess amino acids result in greater level of nitrogen waste for liver and kidneys. Protein needs are proportional to body weight (eg.) large athletes require more protein. Protein supplements are not needed in the American diet.

How much protein do athletes really need?, by P. McCarthy. PHYSICIAN AND SPORTS MEDICINE 17:170-175, MAY 1989
Theoretically, it is possible that large amounts of protein may stimulate growth in muscle mass, but no objective evidence is available. Researchers are studying claims that protein supplements stimulate muscle growth.

How to build muscles. Building bigger, stronger muscles depends on three factors: heredity, exercise and your diet. WRESTLING USA 22(1):8-9, September 20, 1986

Importance of cholesterol control in athletes, by T. Dwyer. EXCEL 3(4):18-20, June 1987

Incompatibility of endurance and strength training modes of exercise, by G. A. Dudley, et al. JOURNAL OF APPLIED PHYSIOLOGY 59(5):1446-1451, November 1985
For this study 14 females and 8 males followed a different training program for 7 weeks: group E trained for endurance, group B for strength, group C for both strength and endurance. Strength training of the knee extensors was done on a isokinetic dynamometer three times a week. Endurance training was done at the same frequency on a cycle ergometer with a work load close to the subjects' peak cycle-ergometer 02 uptake (peak CE VO 2). Tests were performed pre- and post-training and for groups C and E at 14-day intervals as well. The results indicate that concurrent training for strength and endurance reduces the ability to increase muscle strength, whereas strength training does not alter the ability to adapt to endurance training. However, endurance training affects strength development only at fast, not at slow, velocities of contraction.

Influence of protein intake and training status on nitrogen balance and lean body mass, by M. A. Tarnopolsky, et al. JOURNAL OF APPLIED PHYSIOLOGY 64:187-193, 1988
This study examined the effects of training in nitrogen balance, body composition, and urea excretion during periods of habitual and actual protein intakes. Experiments were performed in 6 elite body builders, elite endurance athletes and 6 sedentary controls during a 10-day period of normal protein intake followed by 10-days of altered protein intake. Authors conclude that body builders during habitual training require only slightly greater intake than that for sedentary individuals in the maintenance of lean body mass and that endurance athletes require daily protein intakes greater than either of the other two groups to meet the needs of protein catabolism during exercise.

Internal medicine: safe weight gain, by N. Partin. ATHLETIC TRAINING 22(4): 319+, Winter 1987

This article outlines four steps for safe weight gain and muscle mass without steroids or growth hormones.

Is there a steroid alternative?, R. Pardee . MUSCLE AND FITNESS 45(2):94+, February 1984

Legal performance enhancers: from lion's blood to L-Carnitine, by N. Pena. BICYCLING 28(6):30+, July 1987

Neuromuscular and hormonal responses in elite athletes to two successive strength training sessions in one day, by K. Haekkinen, et al. EUROPEAN JOURNAL OF APPLIED PHYSIOLOGY AND OCCUPATIONAL PHYSI-OLOGY 57(2):133-139, FEBRUARY 1988

Nutritional ergogenic aids: performance boosters?, by L. Houtkooper. SWIMMING WORLD AND JUNIOR SWIMMER 25(10):14-20, October 1984
A nutrition expert sorts out the fact and fiction of the benefits and risks of vitamins and minerals for athletes.

Physiological growth hormone responses of throwers to amino acids, eating and exercise, by P. A. Fricker, et al. AUSTRALIAN JOURNAL OF SCIENCE AND MEDICINE IN SPORT 20(1):21-23, March 1988
Five throwers from the Australian Institute of Sport volunteered to par-ticipate in this study. These athletes undertook a weight training circuit after being assigned to a pre-determined diet and amino acid supplement program. Each athlete took part in six programs (one per week), each program varying with regard to diet, amino acid and placebo intake. The purpose of this study was to investigate the effect of the interaction of diet, amino acid supplements and exercise on the release of growth hormone (GH).

Protein and miscellaneous ergogenic aids, by V. Aronson. PHYSICIAN AND SPORTSMEDICINE 14(5):199-202, May 1986
A nutritionist warns that nutritional supplements can present athletes with some definite risks without guaranteeing benefits. The author, who also wrote about vitamin and mineral supplements in the March 1986 issue, discusses protein supplements, etc. and provides a chart of advertising claims, documented benefits and potential risks. This is an excellent and well-referenced review article.

Protein metabolism related to athletes, by R. Rozenek, et al. NATIONAL STRENGTH AND CONDITIONING ASSOCIATION JOURNAL 6(2):42-45, April/May 1984
This article reviews major aspects of protein metabolism with respect to strength/power type activities, requirements for essential/nonessential amino acids, nitrogen balance and digestion of dietary proteins, RDA fat and carbohydrate requirements, and muscle glycogen and training.

Protein requirements of athletes, by J. R. Brotherhood. EXCEL 3(4):24-26, June 1987

Putting together your strength-training program, by G. Ellis. EXECUTIVE FIT-NESS 16(1):1-2, January 5, 1985

Shocking report: dietary problems of the steroid user, by R. Pardee. MUSCLE AND FITNESS 45(11):72-73+, November 1984

Strength training by resistive exercises, by R. A. Nix. JOURNAL OF THE AR-
KANSAS MEDICAL SOCIETY 82(5):224-227, October 1985

Strength training principles, by M. Kemp. MODERN ATHLETE AND COACH
27(1):3-7, January 1989
Kemp, a coach at the Australia Institute of Sport, presents a detailed
summary of strength development including both principles and
methods used to improve speed strength, strength endurance and
specific strength. Exercises, movements and examples are provided.

Strength training recommendations. AUDIBLE :12, Spring 1986

Sweeping away steroids: nutritional research promises to make drugs obsolete,
by M. Zumpano, et al. MUSCLE AND FITNESS 49(1):124-126, November
1988
Joe Weider promotes his own Victory line of supplements in this article.

Testosterone and growth hormone responses to hypnosis and exercise: a pilot
study, by K. Karpik, et al. NEW ZEALAND JOURNAL OF SPORTS MEDICINE
15(4):88-91, DECEMBER 1987

Tony Pearson's views on the intensity factor, by B. Dobbins. STRENGTH AND
HEALTH 47(2):18-21, February/March 1979
This is a brief article on Mr. America of 1978, Tony Pearson, and his training regimen. Pearson admits having tried anabolic sterodis but never
found he got any benefit.

Tri-iodothyracetic acid abuse in a female body builder, by R. E. Ferner, et al.
LANCET 1(8477):383, February 15, 1986
Brief letter describes 29-year-old female body builder who obtained tri-
iodothyroxine in France. The drug is reported to act on fat to make
muscles appear clearly delineated after a period of high-protein diet,
weight training, and sometimes anabolic steroids and even growth
hormone.

Use of Hungarian milk-protein products in sport, by R. Frenkl, et al. ACTA
MEDICA HUNGARICA 41(2/3):171-173, 1984
Protein-based food products intended for athletes - (Hamomid powder
and tablets, Amino-acid Capsules) - were studied for absorption, elimina-
tion and excretion. On the evidence of the findings, all were readily
absorbed, the serum amino-acid levels attained their peaks 60 to 90
minutes after ingestion of the daily dose. At the end of 10 day periods
in which the products in question had been administered a minor increase was found in the urinary excretion of alpha-aminonitrogen.

Vitamin and mineral status of trained athletes including the effects of supplementation, by L. M. Weight. AMERICAN JOURNAL OF CLINICAL NUTRITION
47(2):186-191, February 1988
Multivitamin and mineral supplementation was without measurable
ergogenic effect and unnecessary in athletes ingesting a normal diet.

Vitamin and mineral supplementation: effect on the running performance of
trained athletes, by L. M. Weight, et al. AMERICAN JOURNAL OF CLINICAL
NUTRITION 47(2):192-195, February 1988
This article reveals that the ingestion of vitamins and minerals . . . exerts
no measurable ergogenic effect.

Vitamins and minerals as ergogenic aids, by V. Aronson. PHYSICIAN AND
SPORTSMEDICINE 14(3):209-212, March 1986

A nutritionist warns that athletes must be on guard against false promises
from nutrient supplements. Author reviews and charts the uses and
abuses of specific vitamins and minerals. Despite the popularity of vitamin
and mineral supplements, performance enhancement has not been
documented except where nutrient deficiencies exist. This is an
excellent overview of the topic with references to books and research
studies.

Vitamins, diet and the athlete, by A. C. Grandjean. CLINICS IN SPORTS MEDI-
CINE 2(1):105-114, March 1983

Optimal nutrition for sport performance can be provided only by sound
dietary habits. While nutritional deficiency can decrease performance,
there is no evidence to suggest that excess consumption beyond normal
requirements is necessary. Toxic effects of some nutrients are discussed.

Women

The effect of anabolic steroids on women is more pronounced than in men because women normally have a much lower testosterone level. Acute side effects are readily seen—weight gain, acne, clitoral enlargement, menstrual irregularity or cessation—and some, such as voice deepening, breast shrinkage, facial and body hair and male pattern baldness, may be irreversible. Women also risk suffering the more serious adverse effects of peliosis hepatitis, reduced serum HDL-cholesterol and hepatocellular carcinoma. This section includes references to both popular and professional articles on physical and emotional problems associated with steroid use by women.

Acute effects of exercise on prolactin and growth hormone secretion: comparison between sedentary women and women runners with normal and abnormal menstrual cycles, by F. E. Chang, et al. JOURNAL OF CLINICAL ENDOCRINOLOGY AND METABOLISM 62(3):551-556, MARCH 1986

Amenorrhea linked to stress of training, competition, by C. E. Haycock. FIRST AIDER 53(7):6-7, Summer 1984
> A major factor in menstrual dysfunction is stress associated with such hormonal changes as the lowering of estrogen levels. The author advises that an athlete be examined by a gynecological endocrinologist if dysfunction occurs.

Anabolic steroid use and perceived effects in ten weight-trained women athletes, by R. H. Strauss, et al. JAMA 253(19):2871-2873, May 17, 1985

Anabolic steroid use by women athletes, by W. N. Taylor, POWERLIFTING USA 8(3):20-21, October 1984

Athletic amenorrhea: an update on aetiology, complications and management, by R. Highet. SPORTS MEDICINE 7(2):82-108, February 1989
> Oligomenorrhoea, primary or secondary amenorrhoea, altered pubertal progression, defective luteal phase, anovulation and infertility may result from those aerobic type activities associated with lower bodyweight and fat percentages such as running, aerobics and gymnastics. Author advises that other causes of amenorrhea not be overlooked in this exercising population and that the diagnosis of "athletic amenorrhoea" not be made until a full thorough history, physical examination and blood tests have eliminated other common causes.

Bodybuilding's apocalypse now, by C. McCloskey. MUSCULAR DEVELOPMENT 24:36-37+, April 1987
> The author feels that the use of steroids in bodybuilding is exaggerated

and has given bodybuilders a bad and undeserved reputation. Random drug testing is recommended.

Characteristics of anabolic-androgenic steroid-free competitive male and female bodybuilders, by D. L. Eliot, et al. PHYSICIAN AND SPORTSMEDICINE 15(6):169-172+, June 1987
Comparison of steroid-free male and female bodybuilders with sedentary controls and runners revealed that the bodybuilders had lower percentages of body fat, probably due to decreased fat stores, stress and alterations in diet and hormone levels. One-third of the female bodybuilders reported menstrual abnormalities. Lipid values of bodybuilders were comparable to a group of lean, aerobically trained athletes.

Chemical use and the woman athlete, K. Donisch Hill. NATIONAL FEDERATION NEWS 3(3):14-15+, 1985
As women's athletics have progressed so have drug usage problems.

Confessions of a steroid user, by D. Barrilleaux. WOMEN'S SPORTS AND FITNESS 9:84, November 1987

Defector says GDR uses steroids, by R. Ingersoll. PHYSICIAN AND SPORTS-MEDICINE 7(3):24-25, March 1979

Drugs and the female athlete: effects . . . side effects . . . after effects, by W. Taylor. MUSCLE AND FITNESS 46:104-107+, September 1985

Effect of anabolic steroids on female athletes, by G. Nevole, et al. ATHLETIC TRAINING 22:297-299, Winter 1987
This review of literature focuses on the female athlete and explores those side effects that may develop.

Exploding the myths: separating facts from fiction, by C. Everson. MUSCLE AND FITNESS 45(7):64-65+, 1984
Bodybuilding: women, men and feminity are among the topics explored in the article.

Female athlete, by R. Jaffe. DELAWARE MEDICAL JOURNAL 59(9):583-586+, September 1987
Increased participation in sports and greater pressures to win have made female athletes very vulnerable to drug abuse. How the physiology and socialization of females contributes to this problem is discussed. This article also reports testing for steroids of first year athletes at the Olympics in 1976. Bodybuilders and powerlifters were found to be heavy users. Use was also prevalent among swimmers and track and field athletes who had not reached full maturity.

Female athletes: targets for drug abuse, by M. Duda. PHYSICIAN AND SPORTS-MEDICINE 14(6):142-146, June 1986

Hormonal alteration in the female athlete, by D. V. Harris. JOURNAL OF DRUG ISSUES 10(3):317-321, Summer 1980
This article briefly discusses the issues of controling the menstrual cycle by oral contraceptives, supplementing with anabolic steroids, inhibiting puberty by "brake" drugs, and transsexualism and sex surgery. These issues are grouped together as hormonal alterations for the purpose of enhancing performance in some sports, but each issue is discussed

56

separately and without comparison or summary. The whole issue is devoted to drugs and sports.

It's not nice to fool Mother Nature, by R. Neufeld. MACLEAN'S 8:31, January 1979

Menstrual irregularity in athletes: basic principles, evaluation and treatment, by M. M. Shangold. CANADIAN JOURNAL OF APPLIED SPORT SCIENCES 7(2): 68-73, June 1982
    During the course of a training program, an athlete may be subjected to many factors including loss of weight and fat, low weight and fat, acute and chronic hormonal changes and physical and emotional stresses. Each of them, alone or in combination, may be associated with menstrual irregularity or amenorrhea. Although these are common problems, the author stresses thorough evaluation of athletes.

Nutritional needs of the female adolescent, by B. L. Morgan, WOMEN AND HEALTH 9(2/3):15-28, Summer-Fall 1984
    The author focuses on the special needs of female adolescent athletes, noting that they require added nutrient intake and a good hydration state for optimal performance.

Pillow talks, by J. Todd. STRENGTH TRAINING FOR BEAUTY 2:65-68, September 1985
    Another woman who openly admits to steroid use is the bodybuilder "Pillow," who began an anti-steroid campaign in 1984.

Rambo drug, by D. Groves. AMERICAN HEALTH 6:43-48, September 1987
    An interview with a former user who won the Ms. America Bodybuilder title in 1982 is featured.

Serum and urinary steroids in women athletes, by J. H. Lukaszewska, et al. JOURNAL OF SPORTS MEDICINE AND PHYSICAL FITNESS 25(4):2-5-221, December 1985

Sleep and growth hormone secretion in women athletes, by B. Walsh, et al. ELECTROENCEPHALOGRAPHY AND CLINICAL NEUROPHYSIOLOGY 57(6):528-531, June 1984
    Six female athletes and five nonathlete controls (aged 20-33 years) underwent 24-hour multiple sampling studies with EEG monitoring of sleep for the assessment of growth hormone secretion and sleep patterns.

Steroids, by M. Shuer. WOMEN'S SPORTS 4(4):17-23+, April 1982
    This author provides an excellent review of steroid use and detection at the olympics and other international competitions from 1956 to 1980. Many female gold medalists and world record holders from the Eastern European countries have tested positive, been suspended, and reinstated to compete very successfully again. Photographs of some of these superwomen from track and field are included. The author also reviews side effects for women athletes and discusses drug testing and ways that athletes beat the tests. Comments from American, Canadian, and two East German defectors verify that female athletes are pressured to use steroids to be bigger, stronger, and faster, especially in swimming and track and field events.

Steroid stand, by J. Ullyot. WOMEN'S SPORTS AND FITNESS 7:10, October
1985
> Brief article in question and answer format on what steroids are and
> examples of different ones.

Straight talking—steroids and the female athlete, by S. Haynes. ACTIVE:
WOMEN IN SPORT NEWSLETTER 2(1):1+, Summer 1989

Strength training for female athletes, by J. Todd. JOURNAL OF PHYSICAL
EDUCATION, RECREATION AND DANCE : 38-39, August 1985

Glossary

ACROMEGALY
  bony overgrowth of skull, facial features, hands, thickening of skin, primarily produced by an oversupply of growth hormone during adulthood

ALOPECIA
  male pattern baldness

AMENORRHEA
  absence of menstruation

ANABOLIC
  tissue-building

ANABOLIC STEROIDS
  synthetic derivatives of testosterone, a natural male sex hormone, used to increase body mass, muscle and strength

ANDROGENIC
  masculinizing, i.e., increased facial hair, deepening voice, etc.

ATHEROGENIC
  producing degeneration in arterial walls, i.e., producing fatty deposits of the inner coat of the arteries (hardening of the arteries)

BODYBUILDERS' PSYCHOSIS
  psychiatric symptoms characterized by hallucinations, self-injury, violence, rage and depression when steroids are discontinued

BRAKE DRUGS
  drugs that retard certain body development, by delaying puberty

CATABOLISM
  any destructive metabolic process by which organisms convert substances into excreted compounds

CHOLESTATIC JAUNDICE
  Inflammation of the liver caused by hepatitis infection. Signs are persistent jaundice, itching, etc., also HEPATIC CHOLESTASIS or CHOLESTASIS, HEPATITIS

CLITEROL HYPERTROPHY
  enlargement of the clitoris, the small organ at the anterior of the vulva homologous to the penis; also CLITOROMEGALY

CORTICOSTEROIDS
group of hormones with cortisone-like action used to combat inflammation or anti-inflammatory

DECA-DURABOLIN
an injected anabolic steroid, a favorite among weight lifters; also taken by Brian Bosworth, University of Oklahoma's all-american linebacker, barred from 1987 Orange Bowl, considered one of the most dangerous because it is administered in an oil-based solution and released over weeks and months and the pituitary is suppressed for a long time.

DIANABOL
trademark for methandro-stanolone; withdrawn from the market by Ciba Geigy in April 1982 due to inappropriate use

DIURETIC
increases the excretion of urine, used to flush drugs from the body before a competition or testing

DOPING
giving or taking an illicit, habit-forming or narcotic drug

DRUG HOLIDAY
remaining drug-free for a period of time

EPIPHYSEAL PLATE
cartilage that separates the head of a long bone and the shaft of the bone; premature closure leads to short stature

ERGOGENIC AID
substance or technique that enhances performance

GIGANTISM
excessive size and stature due to overabundant supply of growth hormone during adolescence

GROWTH HORMONE (GH)
vertebrate polypeptide hormone that stimulates growth, synthetic preparation, growth hormone recombinant, used to treat growth failure in children; undetectable in drug testing; also HUMAN GROWTH HORMONE (HGH)

GYNECOMASTIA
excessive development of male mammary glands or breast enlargement, fairly common side effect in high-dose steroid user

HEPATOMA
liver tumor, sometimes regresses and follows benign course after steroids discontinued, but rapidly fatal in others; linked with long-term high dosages of oral anabolic steroids

HEPATOMEGALY
enlargement of the liver

HEPATOSPLENOMEGALY
coincident enlargement of the liver and spleen

HIRSUTISM
> excessive growth of facial and body hair in women

HUMAN CHORIONIC GONADOTROPIN (HCG)
> chemical component of the urine of pregnent women, sometimes used by male bodybuilders to self-treat gynecomastia; also causes a man's body to produce more testosterone which in turn promotes muscular growth

LIPOPROTEIN
> conjugated protein in which lipids form an integral part, synthesized primarily in the liver, containing various amounts of triglycerides, cholesterol, etc., kinds are high and low density; athletes taking anabolic steroids have changes in blood lipids characteristic of high risk groups for coronary heart disease

MASKING AGENT
> substance that covers or conceals the presence, i.e., PROBENECID used to block the detection of anabolic steroids in urine testing

MEDROXYPROGESTERONE ACETATE
> synthetic drug that is derived from progesterone; thought to be used as a brake drug by communist-bloc female gymnasts

METHANDROSTENOLONE
> androgen and popular anabolic steroid

OLIGOSPERMIA
> scantiness of semen or insufficient spermatozoa in the semen; side effect of anabolic steroid use in male

PLACEBO
> preparation containing no medicine but given for its psychological effect

PELIOSIS HEPATITIS
> abnormal condition characterized by the occurance of numerous small blood-filled cystic lesions throughout the liver which may rupture resulting in hemorrhage or liver failure

PRIAPISM
> abnormal condition of prolonged or constant penile erection, often painful; sometimes side effect of anabolic steroids in young adolescents

ROID RAGES
> term used to describe mood changes that lead to violence and even murder

ROIDS or ROIDALS OR ROID HEADS
> slang names for those who take anabolic steroids (Ben Johnson called, "Benoid.")

SOMATOMEDIN
> group of peptides formed in the liver and other tissues and found in plasma which mediate the effect of growth hormone on cartilage, i.e., growth factors

SOMATOTROPIN: see GROWTH HORMONE

STACKING
> using two or more oral and/or injectable anabolic steroids in different cycles

STACKING THE PYRAMID
> taking several different anabolic steroids in different cycles

STROMBA
> trade name for STANOZOLOL, steroid found in Ben Johnson's urine test

TESTOSTERONE
> male sex hormone; more difficult to detect in drug screening than anabolic steroids

VITAMIN B12
> water-soluble, member of vitamin B complex, cobalt-containing compound that occurs in liver, essential to normal blood function and growth; used in animal feed as a growth factor

VITAMIN B15
> chemical concoction composed of two carcinogens—often known as Paganate or Paganic Acid

Author Index

Brief Subject Index